Obstetric Emergencies

Diogo Ayres-de-Campos

Obstetric Emergencies

A Practical Guide

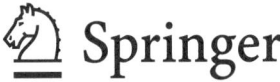

Diogo Ayres-de-Campos
Medical School
University of Porto
Porto
Portugal

ISBN 978-3-319-41654-0   ISBN 978-3-319-41656-4   (eBook)
DOI 10.1007/978-3-319-41656-4

Library of Congress Control Number: 2016951938

© Springer International Publishing Switzerland 2017
This work is subject to copyright. All rights are reserved by the Publisher, whether the whole or part of the material is concerned, specifically the rights of translation, reprinting, reuse of illustrations, recitation, broadcasting, reproduction on microfilms or in any other physical way, and transmission or information storage and retrieval, electronic adaptation, computer software, or by similar or dissimilar methodology now known or hereafter developed.
The use of general descriptive names, registered names, trademarks, service marks, etc. in this publication does not imply, even in the absence of a specific statement, that such names are exempt from the relevant protective laws and regulations and therefore free for general use.
The publisher, the authors and the editors are safe to assume that the advice and information in this book are believed to be true and accurate at the date of publication. Neither the publisher nor the authors or the editors give a warranty, express or implied, with respect to the material contained herein or for any errors or omissions that may have been made.

Printed on acid-free paper

This Springer imprint is published by Springer Nature
The registered company is Springer International Publishing AG Switzerland

Preface

When I started practicing Obstetrics and Gynecology in Porto, some 25 years ago, obstetric emergencies were looked upon by healthcare professionals as events of an almost "supernatural" nature. After such emergencies occurred, people almost invariably put on an expression of fear and fatality. "I pray that this never happens to me when I'm on call" was commonly heard. The occurrence was usually recounted in detail from individual to individual, with some consequent distortion of the facts, and normally very little was learnt from it. Some doctors appeared to be very sure of what should have been done, but opinions frequently differed among them. As a junior doctor at the time, I felt very unsure of what to do should an obstetric emergency happen to me. Memories remain of very stressful cases of acute fetal hypoxia, shoulder dystocia, and postpartum hemorrhage, with many people talking at the same time, contradictory orders and some adverse neonatal and maternal outcomes.

The wide dissemination of evidence-based practice did not do a lot to improve this situation. Acute events are poor candidates for studies providing the highest levels of evidence. Obstetric emergencies were consequently given limited relevance at scientific meetings and medical journals, as there was not a lot of good evidence to discuss, and also because doctors who become well-know in these environments were frequently not involved in the clinical activities where the majority of these situations occur.

The largest contribution to the management of obstetric emergencies over the last decades probably came from the development of clinical guidelines, many of which were based mainly on expert opinion and small case series. Another strong contribution came from the development of more realistic obstetric simulators and the dissemination of simulation-based training courses.

After being involved in the co-ordination of local, national and international guidelines on these subjects, having run simulation-based courses in obstetric emergencies for more than 10 years, and being a medical advisor for the development of a high-fidelity obstetric simulator, I felt the time had come to share some of these experiences in a book. A lot can be learned from observing multiprofessional teams manage obstetric emergencies in the protected environment of simulation, and then formulating an objective and structured way of teaching them to junior doctors. Similar experiences can be gained from developing the requirements of a high-fidelity simulator. Priorities can be reconsidered and the relevance of existing recommendations can be re-evaluated.

With the natural limitation of the quality of existing scientific evidence to support many of the recommendations, I trust that the present book will constitute a useful contribution to healthcare professionals involved in the clinical management of obstetric emergencies, and an opportunity to revise and re-think some of the necessary attitudes.

Contents

1	**Introduction**	1
Part I	**Predominantly Fetal Emergencies**	
2	**Acute Fetal Hypoxia/Acidosis**	7
2.1	Definition, Incidence and Main Risk Factors	7
2.2	Consequences	10
2.3	Diagnosis	10
	2.3.1 Reversible Causes	11
	2.3.1.1 Uterine Hypercontractility	11
	2.3.1.2 Sudden Maternal Hypotension	12
	2.3.1.3 Maternal Supine Position with Aorto-Caval Compression	13
	2.3.2 Irreversible Utero-Placental-Umbilical Disorders	13
	2.3.2.1 Major Placental Abruption	13
	2.3.2.2 Uterine Rupture	14
	2.3.2.3 Umbilical Cord Prolapse	15
	2.3.3 Maternal Cardiorespiratory Disorders	16
	2.3.4 Usually Occult Causes	16
	2.3.4.1 Occult Cord Compression	16
	2.3.4.2 Major Fetal Haemorrhage	17
	2.3.5 Specific Mechanical Complications of Labour	18
2.4	Clinical Management	18
	2.4.1 Immediate Actions in Face of a Prolonged Deceleration	18
	2.4.2 Uterine Hypercontractility	20
	2.4.3 Sudden Maternal Hypotension	20
	2.4.4 Major Placental Abruption	21
	2.4.5 Uterine Rupture	21
	2.4.6 Umbilical Cord Prolapse	22
	2.4.7 Maximum Time Limits for Reversal of a Prolonged Deceleration	22
2.5	Clinical Records and Litigation Issues	23

3 Shoulder Dystocia 27
- 3.1 Definition, Incidence and Main Risk Factors 27
- 3.2 Complications 29
- 3.3 Diagnosis 31
- 3.4 Clinical Management 31
  - 3.4.1 Anticipating the Situation 31
  - 3.4.2 Clearly Verbalising the Diagnosis 32
  - 3.4.3 Avoiding Manoeuvres That Increase the Risk of Fetal Injury 32
  - 3.4.4 Asking for Help 32
  - 3.4.5 External Manoeuvres 32
  - 3.4.6 Internal Manoeuvres 33
  - 3.4.7 All-Fours Manoeuvre (Gaskin's Manoeuvre) ... 35
  - 3.4.8 Exceptional Manoeuvres 36
- 3.5 Clinical Records and Litigation Issues 37

4 Retention of the After-Coming Head 41
- 4.1 Definition, Incidence and Main Risk Factors 41
- 4.2 Consequences 42
- 4.3 Diagnosis 43
- 4.4 Clinical Management 43
  - 4.4.1 Guaranteeing the Conditions for a Safe Vaginal Breech Delivery 43
  - 4.4.2 Anticipate the Situation 44
  - 4.4.3 Attempts to Deliver the Fetal Head 44
  - 4.4.4 Clearly Verbalising the Diagnosis 45
  - 4.4.5 Asking for Help 45
  - 4.4.6 McRobert's Position 46
  - 4.4.7 Episiotomy 46
  - 4.4.8 Fetal Monitoring 46
  - 4.4.9 Insertion of a Vaginal Retractor 46
  - 4.4.10 Forceps to the After-Coming Head 46
  - 4.4.11 Exceptional Manoeuvres 48
- 4.5 Clinical Records and Litigation Issues 48

Part II Predominantly Maternal Emergencies

5 Eclampsia 53
- 5.1 Definition, Incidence and Main Risk Factors 53
- 5.2 Complications 54
- 5.3 Diagnosis 54
- 5.4 Clinical Management 54
  - 5.4.1 Anticipate and Prevent the Situation 54
  - 5.4.2 Ask for Help 55
  - 5.4.3 Avoid Lesions During the Eclamptic Seizure .. 55

		5.4.4	Left Lateral Safety Position, Inspect Airway and Monitor	55
		5.4.5	Prevention of New Seizures	56
		5.4.6	Other Non-emergent Measures	56
		5.4.7	Decreasing Blood Pressure	56
		5.4.8	Recurrent Seizures	57
		5.4.9	Maintenance Dose of Magnesium Sulphate	58
		5.4.10	Fluid Balance	59
		5.4.11	Thromboprophylaxis	59
		5.4.12	Evaluation of Laboratory Results and Fetal Evaluation	59
		5.4.13	Programming Birth	59
	5.5	Clinical Records and Litigation Issues		60
6	**Postpartum Haemorrhage**			63
	6.1	Definition, Incidence and Main Risk Factors		63
	6.2	Consequences		66
	6.3	Diagnosis		66
	6.4	Clinical Management		66
		6.4.1	Anticipating the Situation	66
		6.4.2	Clearly Verbalising the Diagnosis	67
		6.4.3	Asking for Help	67
		6.4.4	Initial Evaluation of the Cause of Haemorrhage	67
		6.4.5	Support of Maternal Circulation and Oxygenation	67
			6.4.5.1 Venous Catheterisation and Blood Volume Replacement	67
			6.4.5.2 Maternal Monitoring	68
			6.4.5.3 Bladder Catheterisation and Measurement of Urinary Output	68
			6.4.5.4 Maintain Maternal Oxygen Supply to the Brain	68
			6.4.5.5 Decision to Start Colloids	68
			6.4.5.6 Decision to Administer Blood Products	68
			6.4.5.7 Maintain Body Temperature	69
		6.4.6	Treatment of Uterine Atony	69
			6.4.6.1 Initial Measures	69
			6.4.6.2 Medical Treatment	69
			6.4.6.3 Mechanical Treatments	70
			6.4.6.4 Surgical Treatments	71
			6.4.6.5 Pelvic Tamponade	74
		6.4.7	Treatment of Birth Canal Injuries	74
		6.4.8	Treatment of Placental Retention	76
			6.4.8.1 Complete Placental Retention	76
			6.4.8.2 Partial Placental Retention	76
		6.4.9	Treatment of Rare Causes of Postpartum Haemorrhage	76
			6.4.9.1 Uterine Inversion	76

		6.4.9.2	Uterine Rupture	77
		6.4.9.3	Abnormally Adherent Placenta	77
		6.4.9.4	Maternal Bleeding Disorders	78
	6.4.10		Postpartum Haemorrhage at Caesarean Section	78
6.5	Clinical Records and Litigation Issues			78

7 Maternal Cardiorespiratory Arrest 81

- 7.1 Definition, Incidence and Main Risk Factors 81
- 7.2 Consequences 82
- 7.3 Diagnosis 82
- 7.4 Clinical Management 82
  - 7.4.1 Anticipating the Situation 82
  - 7.4.2 Clearly Verbalising the Diagnosis 82
  - 7.4.3 Asking for Help 83
  - 7.4.4 Maternal Monitoring 83
  - 7.4.5 Support of Maternal Oxygenation and Circulation 83
    - 7.4.5.1 A (Airway): Guarantee the Patency of the Airway 83
    - 7.4.5.2 B (Breathing): Maintain Oxygen Supply to the Lungs ... 83
    - 7.4.5.3 C (Circulation): Cardiac Massage and Vein Catheterisation 84
  - 7.4.6 Bladder Catheterisation and Measurement of Urinary Output 85
  - 7.4.7 Fetal Monitoring 85
  - 7.4.8 *In Situ* Caesarean Section 85
  - 7.4.9 Defibrillatory Rhythms 85
  - 7.4.10 After Cardiorespiratory Arrest Reverses 86
    - 7.4.10.1 Hypotension 86
    - 7.4.10.2 Termination of Pregnancy 86
    - 7.4.10.3 Monitoring in an Intensive Care Unit ... 87
    - 7.4.10.4 Maintain Body Temperature 87
    - 7.4.10.5 Looking for an Underlying Cause ... 87
  - 7.4.11 Pulmonary Thromboembolism 87
  - 7.4.12 Amniotic Fluid Embolism Syndrome 88
- 7.5 Clinical Records and Litigation Issues 89

Introduction

Obstetrics is a unique area of healthcare, in that the vast majority of situations in pregnancy and childbirth have normal outcome, even when there is no intervention from healthcare professionals. However, serious complications do occur in a smaller number of cases, and increased knowledge on their diagnosis and treatment has made a tremendous difference to maternal and fetal outcomes over the last 200 years. One could even say that obstetrics is somewhat a victim of its own success, as improvements have been so striking that much of society has erroneously perceived adverse outcomes to have disappeared and, when they occur, frequently judges them to be due to malpractice.

Progress achieved over the last decades in high-resource countries has resulted in marked decreases in maternal and perinatal mortality. In the last 80 years, maternal mortality decreased almost a 100-fold in many European countries, to values that are currently between 5 and 10 per 100,000 births. Perinatal mortality also decreased more than tenfold, to values between 3 and 10 per 1000 births. Equally important, but less well documented, is the decrease in long-term maternal and child morbidity consequent to the complications of pregnancy and childbirth.

In spite of the unquestionable success of modern obstetrical care in reducing the burden of disease associated with the reproductive process, there is still margin for improvement. According to confidential enquiries into maternal and perinatal deaths carried out over the last two decades in the United Kingdom, substandard care continues to be identified in around 50 % of cases.

Healthcare professionals working in moderate-sized European centres usually maintain experience in management of most obstetric situations by literature review and day-to-day clinical practice, but rare situations exist where lack of familiarity with the clinical entity causes apprehension and uncertainty. Some of these situations are not acute in nature, so they allow time for consultation of the literature, but others require immediate action in order to guarantee a positive outcome. These are the most feared, and sometimes even healthcare professionals with decades of experience in obstetrical care have limited practice in their management.

Acute complications of pregnancy and childbirth, posing risk to the mother and/or the fetus, and whose resolution requires an almost immediate response from the healthcare team (usually in a few minutes) in order to guarantee a favourable outcome – this is the concept that best describes **obstetric emergencies**.

Resolution of these situations not only requires a thorough **knowledge** of their diagnosis and management but also specific **technical skills** (in this case manual skills) that because of reduced exposure are difficult to learn and to maintain competence. Unless healthcare professionals regularly attend simulation-based courses, most find it difficult to retain proficiency, for instance, in executing internal manoeuvres for the resolution of shoulder dystocia, applying forceps to the after-coming head, executing the Zavanelli manoeuvre or symphysiotomy or inserting a Bakri balloon.

Management of these situations usually requires the collaboration between multiple professionals within a healthcare team, so **teamwork skills** are also important. The latter includes the capacity of a team member to assume **leadership** and to hand it over when a more experienced person arrives, as well as the capacity of the remaining team to cooperate with the leader. Inherent to these concepts are the skills for **adequate task distribution**, **feedback** and **support** between team members. **Communication skills** assume a central role in all of these aspects, not only for the interactions between healthcare professionals but also with patients and their families.

Finally, it should not be forgotten that **organisational aspects** of healthcare facilities may also play a part in the resolution of these situations. Ease of contact and timely availability of healthcare professionals are crucial for successful management, as is the accessibility to clinical materials and the guarantee of their usability.

Given the rarity of these situations, the social burden of adverse outcomes and the difficulty in maintaining adequate clinical competence, **simulation-based training courses in obstetric emergencies**, initially developed in the United States and United Kingdom in the 1990s, have been introduced in many European countries. These courses use patient actors and a new generation of obstetric simulators developed over the last two decades, to allow realistic and interactive multiprofessional team training.

Regular attendance of such courses has become a routine part of training and accreditation in many centres, and there is data to suggest that it is associated with reduced incidence of adverse perinatal outcomes, including brachial plexus injury and hypoxic-ischaemic encephalopathy.

This book provides a practical guide to the diagnosis and management of obstetric emergencies. It can be used for review and consultation of specific clinical procedures, and it is also a useful reference manual for simulation-based courses. The topics covered include "predominately fetal" emergencies – acute fetal hypoxia/acidosis, shoulder dystocia, and retention of the after-coming head; as well as "predominately maternal" emergencies – eclampsia, cardiorespiratory arrest, and postpartum haemorrhage.

Suggested Reading

Black RS, Brocklehurst P (2003) A systematic review of training in acute obstetric emergencies. BJOG 110:837–841

CEMACH (2006) Confidential enquiry into maternal and child health. Perinatal mortality surveillance 2004: England, Wales and Northern Ireland. CEMACH, London

CEMACH (2007) Saving mothers' lives 2003–2005. CEMACH, London

CESDI (1997) Confidential enquiry into stillbirths and deaths in infancy. 4th annual report. Maternal and Child Health Research Consortium, London

Draycott TJ, Sibanda T, Owen L, Akande V, Winter C, Reading S, Whitelaw A (2006) Does training in obstetric emergencies improve neonatal outcome? BJOG 113:177–182

Draycott TJ, Crofts JF, Ash JP, Wilson LV, Yard E, Sibanda T, Whitelaw A (2008) Improving neonatal outcome through practical shoulder dystocia training. Obstet Gynecol 112:14–20

World Health Organization (2006) Neonatal and perinatal mortality: country, regional and global estimates. WHO Press, Geneva

Part I
Predominantly Fetal Emergencies

Acute Fetal Hypoxia/Acidosis

2.1 Definition, Incidence and Main Risk Factors

Fetal hypoxia refers to the condition in which there is decreased oxygen concentration in fetal tissues, and this is insufficient to maintain normal cell energy production by way of aerobic metabolism. Oxygen is supplied to fetal tissues via a long pathway that involves the maternal respiratory system, maternal circulation, gas exchange at the placenta and finally the umbilical and fetal circulations (Fig. 2.1). Problems occurring at any of these levels may result in decreased oxygen concentration in the fetal circulation (hypoxaemia) and ultimately in fetal tissues (hypoxia).

Acute fetal hypoxia refers to the condition in which there is a rapid reduction in oxygen levels, i.e. occurring over the course of a few minutes. Its main causes are considered in Table 2.1.

In the absence of oxygen, fetal cells may continue to produce the energy required for maintenance of basic homeostatic functions during a few more minutes, by resorting to **anaerobic metabolism**. However, the latter yields much less energy than aerobic metabolism and results in the production of lactic acid. The intra- and extracellular accumulation of hydrogen ions, due to increased lactic acid production, results in the development of **metabolic acidosis** (decreased pH caused by acids of intracellular origin) and, because these ions are taken away by the fetal circulation, metabolic acidaemia. The whole process of decreased oxygen concentration in tissues is therefore known as **hypoxia/acidosis**.

Some constituents of fetal blood are capable of neutralising (buffering) hydrogen ions. These are called **bases**, and they include bicarbonate, haemoglobin and plasma proteins. However, their availability is limited, and their depletion (**base deficit**) is directly related to the severity of metabolic acidosis. As there is no direct method of quantifying oxygen concentration within fetal tissues, the only objective way of diagnosing intrapartum fetal hypoxia/acidosis is to measure pH and base deficit in the umbilical cord blood at delivery or in the newborn circulation during the first minutes of life. Metabolic acidosis is defined as a pH below 7.00 and a base deficit in excess of 12 mmol/l (or alternatively a lactate value in excess of 10 mmol/l) in

Fig. 2.1 A representation of the pathway of oxygen supply to the fetus

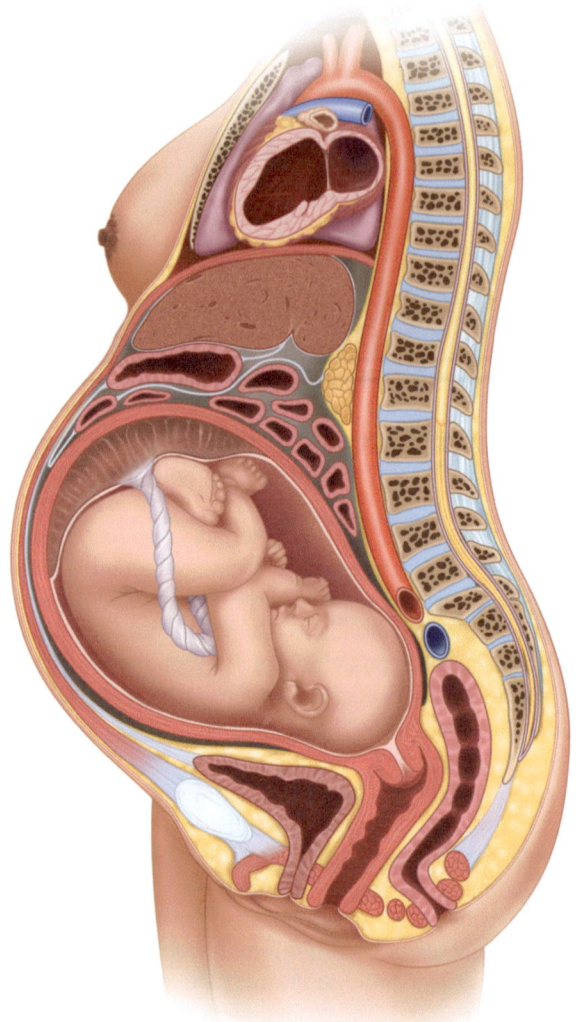

either of these circulations. The umbilical cord does not need to be clamped for sampling, but it is important to obtain blood from both artery and vein as soon as possible after birth, to guarantee the quality of results. Sampling of the wrong vessel may occur when the needle crosses the artery to pierce the vein, and this may also result in mixed sampling. After blood is drawn into two heparinised syringes, existing air bubbles are removed and the syringes capped and rolled between the fingers to mix blood with heparin; blood gas analysis should be performed within the next

Table 2.1 Main causes of acute fetal hypoxia/acidosis

Reversible causes
Uterine hypercontractility
Sudden maternal hypotension
Maternal supine position with aorto-caval compression
Irreversible causes
Major placental abruption
Uterine rupture
Umbilical cord prolapse
Maternal cardiorespiratory disorders
Severe asthma, haemorrhagic shock, cardiorespiratory arrest, pulmonary thromboembolism, amniotic fluid embolism, generalised seizures, etc.
Usually occult causes
Occult cord compression (true cord knot, low-lying cord, nuchal cord with stretching)
Major fetal haemorrhage (fetal-maternal haemorrhage, ruptured vasa praevia)
Specific mechanical complications of labour
Shoulder dystocia
Retention of the after-coming head

30 min. When the difference in pH between the two samples is less than 0.02 and the difference in pCO_2 is less than 5 mmHg (0.7 Kilopascal), samples are likely to be mixed or to have been obtained from the same vessel. When hypoxia/acidosis is of acute onset, there is usually also a large difference in pH between artery and vein.

Increasing concentrations of hydrogen ions that are no longer buffered because of base depletion affect energy production and cell homeostasis, leading to disrupted cell function and ultimately to a cascade of biochemical events that results in cell death. When hypoxia is sufficiently intense and prolonged to disrupt neurological, respiratory and cardiovascular control, this is reflected in reduced **Apgar scores** at birth. Apgar scores however are much less specific indicators of fetal hypoxia than umbilical blood gas values, as they can be affected by other factors such as prematurity, central nervous system depressors administered to the mother, birth trauma without hypoxia (i.e., subdural haematoma), infection, meconium aspiration, congenital anomalies, pre-existing lesions and early neonatal interventions such as vigorous endotracheal aspiration.

The overall incidence of fetal hypoxia/acidosis, as defined by the incidence of newborn metabolic acidosis, varies substantially between different European hospitals, depending on the risk characteristics of the population and on labour management strategies. Reported rates vary between 0.06 and 2.8 %.

The major risk factors for acute fetal hypoxia/acidosis are the ones responsible for its underlying causes: i.e. labour induction and augmentation with prostaglandins or oxytocin are major risk factors for uterine hypercontractility, regional analgesia is a major risk factor for sudden maternal hypotension, and early amniotomy is a risk factor for uterine hypercontractility and umbilical cord prolapse. A detailed description of the risk factors for all causes of acute fetal hypoxia/acidosis is beyond the aim of this book.

2.2 Consequences

Most newborns with metabolic acidosis and low Apgars recover quickly and do not develop short- or long-term functional impairments. However, when fetal hypoxia/acidosis is sufficiently intense and prolonged, changes in neurological function may become apparent in the first 48 h of life, manifested by hypotonia, seizures and/or coma, a situation that is termed **hypoxic-ischaemic encephalopathy**. In its mild forms (grade 1), a short period of hypotonia is documented, but very rarely it evolves into permanent handicap. When the newborn develops seizures (grade 2), the risk of mortality or long-term neurological sequelae is about 20–30 %. When a comatose state occurs (grade 3), perinatal death or long-term handicap is frequent.

Not all cases of neurological dysfunction occurring in the first 48 h of life (neonatal encephalopathy) are caused by fetal hypoxia/acidosis, so to establish the diagnosis of hypoxic-ischaemic encephalopathy, it is necessary to document metabolic acidosis in the umbilical cord or in the newborn circulation in the first minutes of life.

Cerebral palsy of the dyskinetic or spastic quadriplegic types is the long-term neurological sequela most strongly associated with fetal hypoxia/acidosis, although only 10–20 % of cases are caused by this entity. Perinatal infection, congenital diseases, metabolic diseases, coagulation disorders and the complications associated with birth trauma and prematurity constitute the majority of causal factors.

The speed of installation and intensity of acute fetal hypoxia/acidosis varies from case to case, so fetal risk is not uniform. In some cases, there may be a sudden and almost total reduction in oxygen supply, while in others, it may be less intense or of slower onset. The insults can also be transitory and repetitive in nature (uterine hypercontractility, occult cord compression). Finally, there is also some individual variation in the capacity to react to hypoxia/acidosis.

For all these reasons, it is difficult to establish how long a hypoxic insult may last before important injury occurs. However, some information can be extrapolated from cases of sudden maternal cardiorespiratory arrest. No long-term neurological sequelae were reported when the interval between arrest and birth was under 12 min, and perinatal death was common when more than 15 min had elapsed. This evidence is frequently used as an indicator of a 12-min margin of safety for the fetus, in situations where sudden and complete interruption of fetal oxygenation occurs. It is likely that this rule of thumb is only valid for normally grown fetuses at term, receiving adequate oxygenation before the insult occurred, and needs to be adapted in other situations.

2.3 Diagnosis

Acute fetal hypoxia/acidosis almost always manifests as a **prolonged deceleration** – a sudden and sustained decrease in the fetal heart rate (FHR), with an amplitude exceeding 15 bpm and lasting more than 3 min (Fig. 2.2). When the duration exceeds 10 min, it is called **fetal bradycardia**.

2.3 Diagnosis

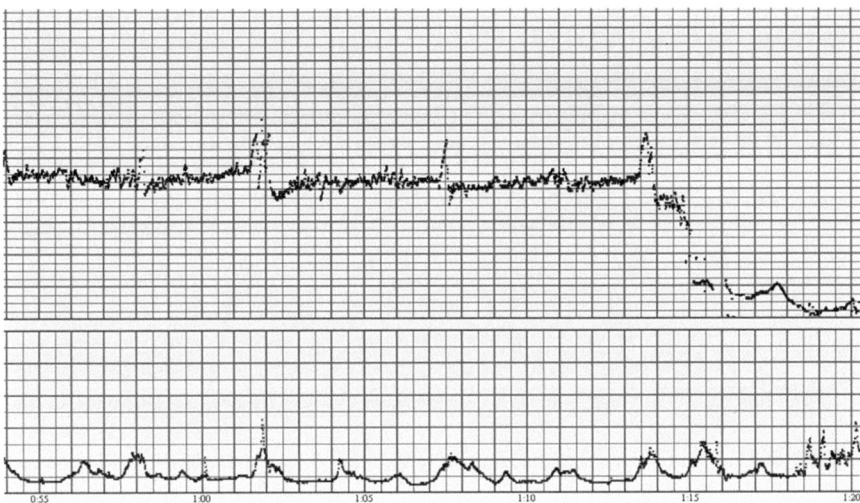

Fig. 2.2 Cardiotocographic (CTG) tracing with prolonged FHR deceleration and reduced variability within the deceleration ("paper speed" 1 cm/min)

Decreased oxygen concentration in fetal arterial blood triggers chemoreceptors located near the aortic arch to transmit neurological impulses to brain stem nuclei controlling the vagus nerve and causes a parasympathetically mediated drop in FHR. When fetal hypoxia/acidosis affects the central nervous system, the sympathetic-parasympathetic modulation of FHR is decreased, and this results in diminished signal oscillations, a phenomenon known as **reduced variability** (Fig. 2.2).

Other clinical symptoms and signs may appear in association with a prolonged deceleration, related to the underlying cause of fetal hypoxia/acidosis (see below).

2.3.1 Reversible Causes

The underlying cause of fetal hypoxia/acidosis is frequently reversible, as occurs with uterine hypercontractility, sudden maternal hypotension or aorto-caval compression by the pregnant uterus when the mother is in the supine position.

2.3.1.1 Uterine Hypercontractility
Uterine contractions compress the blood vessels running inside the myometrium, and this may cause a temporary reduction in placental perfusion. The umbilical cord may also be compressed between fetal bony parts or between the fetal head and the uterine wall, transitorily reducing umbilical blood flow. Usually these phenomena occur during the peak of uterine contractions, and the intervals between these events are sufficient to re-establish normal oxygenation. The frequency, duration and intensity of uterine contractions will determine the magnitude of the disturbances, and how much they affect fetal oxygenation.

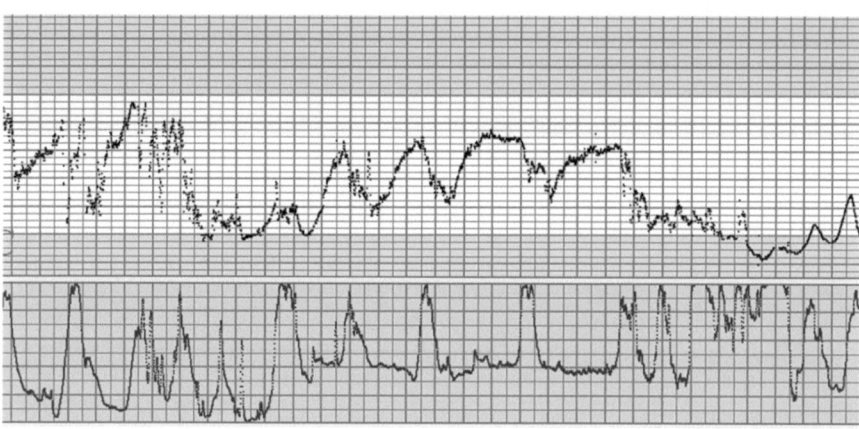

Fig. 2.3 CTG with uterine hypercontractility (tachysystole), prolonged decelerations with attempts to recover between contractions and reduced variability at the end ("paper speed" 1 cm/min)

Hypercontractility may be spontaneous or induced in nature and refers to an increased frequency, intensity and/or duration of contractions leading to reduced fetal oxygenation. Rather than exhibiting a single prolonged deceleration (Fig. 2.2), uterine hypercontractility usually manifests by repetitive decelerations that may merge to become a prolonged deceleration and ultimately exhibit loss of variability but with a tendency for FHR recovery between contractions (Fig. 2.3).

Most cases of uterine hypercontractility are iatrogenic in nature, caused by oxytocin or prostaglandin administration. Local practices for labour induction and acceleration will therefore determine the incidence of this entity, and respecting established doses and intervals for drug administration limits its occurrence. Little is known about the incidence and risk factors of spontaneous uterine hypercontractility, but some cases have been described in association with myometrial infection and partial placental abruption.

Increased abdominal pain is usually referred, but in the context of epidural analgesia, the diagnosis will rely mainly on the detection of increased contraction frequency by cardiotocography (CTG) or on uterine fundus palpation. More than five contractions in 10 min on two successive 10-min periods or averaged in the last 30 min is the definition of **tachysystole** – increased frequency of uterine contractions. With external monitoring of uterine contractions, using a tocodynamometer or fundal palpation, only frequency of uterine contractions can be reliability assessed. Evaluation of their intensity and duration, as well as of basal uterine tone, requires the use of an intrauterine pressure sensor, a technique that is nowadays seldomly used. A sustained rise in uterine contraction baseline or the detection of a permanently contracted uterine fundus is very suggestive of increased basal tone (hypertonus), but intrauterine pressure measurement remains the gold standard for this diagnosis.

2.3.1.2 Sudden Maternal Hypotension

Sudden maternal hypotension is nearly always an iatrogenic complication associated with epidural or spinal analgesia, due to blocking of sympathetic nerves that regulate vessel tonus. It can manifest by nausea, dizziness, vomiting, blurred vision and loss of consciousness and is usually accompanied by a prolonged deceleration. The drop in blood pressure is usually moderate but sufficient to cause a decrease in placental perfusion and gas exchange.

When epidural analgesia began to be used in labour, maternal hypotension and the resulting CTG changes occurred in almost a third of cases. Prophylactic fluid administration before catheter placement reduced this incidence to about 2 %, and recent developments in the technique with lower doses of local anaesthetics have almost eliminated the need for prophylactic fluid administration.

2.3.1.3 Maternal Supine Position with Aorto-Caval Compression

Adoption of the maternal supine position can lead to important aorto-caval compression by the pregnant uterus, with a resulting reduction in placental perfusion and gas exchange. This position has also been associated with uterine hypercontractility due to sacral plexus stimulation. Asking the mother to adopt the upright, half-sitting or lateral recumbent position is usually followed by normalisation of the CTG pattern.

2.3.2 Irreversible Utero-Placental-Umbilical Disorders

These are rare events of an irreversible nature that pose great risk to fetal oxygenation. They include major placental abruption, uterine rupture and umbilical cord prolapse. All of them require rapid delivery to avoid adverse perinatal outcome, and the first two can also be associated with profuse maternal haemorrhage.

2.3.2.1 Major Placental Abruption

Major placental abruption can be defined as a separation between the chorion and decidua of sufficient area to condition fetal oxygenation and/or is associated with maternal haemorrhage of sufficient volume to produce the same effect (Fig. 2.4).

Placental abruption affects about 1 % of all labours, but the vast majority of cases are insidious and of small dimension. Placental function needs to be reduced by about 50 % before fetal oxygenation is affected. Blood originating from vessels located behind the placenta may detach the fetal membranes and drain to the vagina, or it may accumulate to form a retroplacental haematoma. Occasionally, blood will infiltrate the myometrium and originate a Couvelaire uterus, a structure of petrous consistency that can be palpated through the abdomen when located anteriorly and/or fundally.

The main risk factors for placental abruption are a previous history of similar episodes, hypertensive diseases of pregnancy, abdominal trauma, maternal cocaine consumption, maternal smoking and fetal growth restriction.

Sudden abdominal pain, abdominal tenderness, vaginal bleeding and maternal haemodynamic changes may be present, but frequently the first manifestation is a prolonged deceleration. FHR sounds have been reported to be dulled when there is a large anterior placental haematoma, and in these cases it may be necessary to confirm heart movements on ultrasound. When the presenting part is fully engaged, blood may not exteriorise through the vagina and will accumulate inside the uterine cavity, draining after birth.

Fig. 2.4 Major placental abruption

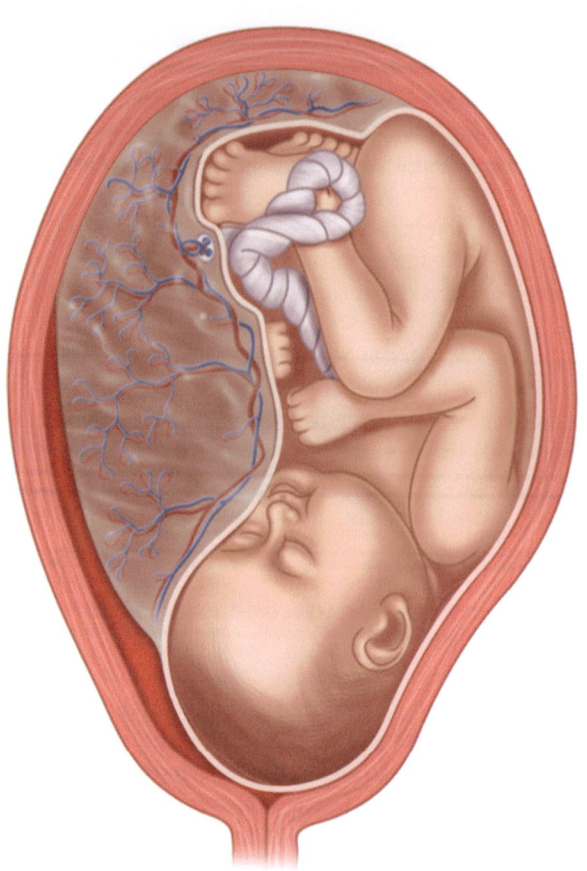

Uterine contractility may be increased in small placental detachments, but in major abruption, it is generally irregular and inefficient, predisposing to postpartum uterine atony. Myometrial infiltration causes the release of thromboplastins into the maternal circulation and may result in disseminated intravascular coagulation.

2.3.2.2 Uterine Rupture

Only about 30 % of cases of uterine rupture are associated with fetal hypoxia/acidosis, because lacerations are frequently limited to the caesarean section scar and do not involve important myometrial vessels irrigating the placental bed nor is there an accompanying major abruption. Acute hypoxia/acidosis is more frequent when the fetus is exteriorised into the peritoneal cavity. Maternal mortality associated with uterine rupture is currently low in high-resource countries. On the other hand, there is a relatively high rate of peripartum hysterectomy.

Uterine rupture affects about 0.003 % of all births, and the incidence does not appear to have increased over the last decades. In the majority of cases, there is a previous history of caesarean section, and the incidence in this population is about 0.1%. Other risk factors include high multiparity, uterine malformations, oxytocin or prostaglandin use, forceps delivery, placenta percreta, external cephalic version, fetal macrosomia, fetal-pelvic disproportion, abnormal fetal presentation and previous uterine surgery, including curettage and hysteroscopy.

Continuous lower abdominal quadrant pain (3–50%) and vaginal bleeding (8–12%) are the most suggestive symptoms of uterine rupture, but a prolonged deceleration (70%) is frequently the only manifestation. Upward displacement of the presenting part has been reported, but does not seem to be frequent nor is it easy to recognise. Sometimes the diagnosis is only apparent at the time of surgery, where caesarean section scar dehiscence is the most frequent finding. Uterine rupture may extend anteriorly to affect the posterior bladder wall or laterally towards the broad ligaments and the uterine arteries, in the latter case causing severe haemorrhage. Extension to the posterior uterine wall is rare in the absence of previous uterine surgery.

Adherence to established guidelines for labour induction and acceleration and continuous FHR monitoring in women with previous uterine scars are required for avoiding and/or rapidly detecting these situations.

2.3.2.3 Umbilical Cord Prolapse

Umbilical cord prolapse is defined as the presence of a loop of umbilical cord below the presenting part, after the membranes have ruptured. The loop usually passes through the cervix into the vagina (Fig. 2.5), but it can also remain in the uterine cavity or pass through the vaginal introitus to the exterior.

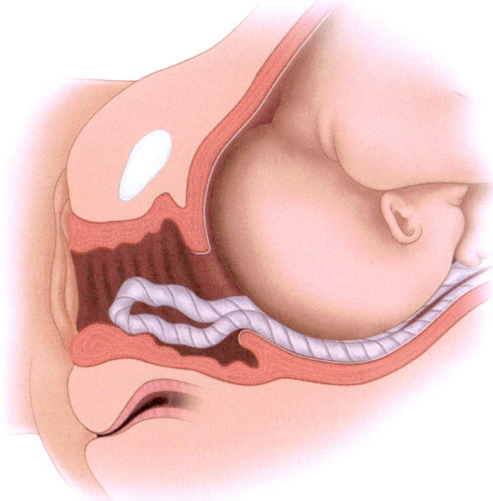

Fig. 2.5 Umbilical cord prolapse

With umbilical cord prolapse, the loop may be continuously compressed between the presenting part and the maternal pelvis, but it can also only be subject to intermittent compressions during contractions. Rarely, no cord compression occurs, a situation that is more frequent with earlier gestational ages, anomalous fetal presentations and in the absence of labour. Cord prolapse can also be complicated by vascular spasm, which has been described when the cord is exposed to cold or is manipulated. During labour, umbilical cord prolapse is almost always associated with repetitive decelerations or with a prolonged deceleration.

Umbilical cord prolapse is reported to affect 0.1–0.6% of all labours, but the incidence may reach 1% in breech presentations. Older studies report severe fetal hypoxia/acidosis to occur in 25–50% of cases, but this number has been decreasing in the last decades, probably due to increased awareness, faster diagnosis and management. Recent studies report perinatal mortality rates between 3.6 and 16.2%, with causes of death more related to prematurity than to fetal hypoxia/acidosis.

The main risk factors for umbilical cord prolapse are anomalous fetal presentations (transverse lie, knee or footling breech), polyhydramnios, multiparity, long umbilical cord, multiple gestation, preterm labour and low-lying placenta. In a recent case series, 47% of cases were preceded by an obstetrical intervention such as amniotomy, fetal electrode placement, intrauterine pressure sensor placement and external cephalic version or by expectant management of preterm premature rupture of membranes.

2.3.3 Maternal Cardiorespiratory Disorders

Fetal hypoxia/acidosis may be caused by a number of acute maternal circulatory and respiratory disorders, including severe asthma, haemorrhagic shock, and cardiorespiratory arrest. During labour, however, the most common causes are pulmonary thromboembolism and amniotic fluid embolism. A more detailed description of these complications is provided in Chap. 7.

2.3.4 Usually Occult Causes

It is not always possible to diagnose the causes of a prolonged deceleration before birth, as there is no clear symptom or sign pointing to an aetiology. The occult causes of acute fetal hypoxia/acidosis include occult cord compression and major fetal haemorrhage.

2.3.4.1 Occult Cord Compression

Occult cord compression may occur because of a tight umbilical cord knot, a low-lying loop compressed by the fetal head or a tight nuchal cord that is stretched during descent of the fetal head. Different degrees of compression may occur, resulting in varying levels of circulatory compromise. In the majority of situations, decreased fetal oxygenation and the accompanying FHR changes only occur during contractions, and the intervals between these events are sufficient to recover fetal oxygenation. The diagnosis is usually retrospective and established at the time of vaginal delivery or caesarean section, but even there low-lying loops may be missed. Depending on the degree of circulatory compromise during and in between contractions, the situation may be relieved by acute tocolysis and by positioning the mother on the left or right lateral, half-sitting or upright positions.

2.3.4.2 Major Fetal Haemorrhage

Fetal haemorrhage of sufficient volume to result in reduced oxygen transport capacity may be chronic, acute or recurring in nature and can be due to fetal-maternal haemorrhage, ruptured vasa praevia or very rarely to lacerations of an umbilical or placental vessel.

In almost all deliveries, there is some degree of **fetal-maternal haemorrhage**, but this is usually of small quantity. A fetal-maternal haemorrhage of more than 20 ml is reported to occur in 0.46 % of births, more than 30 ml in 0.38 % and more than 80 ml in 0.07 %. An increased risk of adverse perinatal outcome is found when blood loss exceeds 20 ml/kg of fetal weight, and about two-thirds of newborns die when it exceeds 80 ml/kg. Other important factors to establish fetal prognosis are the rate of haemorrhage and gestational age. Major fetal-maternal haemorrhage can follow abdominal trauma, external cephalic version, amniocentesis and abruption, and it can also occur with placental chorioangiomas. The vast majority of cases however arise spontaneously and have no identifiable cause. Fetal-maternal haemorrhage is usually asymptomatic, although decreased fetal movements may be reported. The volume of fetal blood present in the maternal circulation should be estimated by the Kleihauer-Betke test or by flow cytometry, and newborn anaemia needs to be documented after birth. Rarely, in the presence of massive haemorrhage, the mother experiences a transfusion reaction with nausea, oedema, chills and fever.

Ruptured vasa praevia refers to the laceration of fetal vessels coursing through the membranes close to the internal cervical *os*, during spontaneous or artificial rupture of membranes. It can occur because of velamentous insertion of the cord or because of vessels running between lobes in a bilobed placenta. The reported incidence is 0.017–0.05 %. Perinatal mortality rate appears to be around 60 % when the situation is diagnosed at membrane rupture, but it can be reduced to 3 % when antenatal diagnosis is followed by elective caesarean section. Ruptured vasa praevia usually presents with vaginal haemorrhage at the time of membrane rupture. Very occasionally the vessels may be palpated on vaginal examination before rupture occurs, and their presence confirmed with transvaginal Doppler ultrasound or with an amnioscope. Risk factors for vasa praevia include bilobed placenta, low-lying placenta diagnosed in the second trimester, multiple pregnancy and in vitro fertilisation.

In major fetal haemorrhage of any cause, a sinusoidal FHR pattern is frequently detected (Fig. 2.6), occasionally with fetal tachycardia during the acute phase, recurrent late decelerations appearing when contractions start or a prolonged deceleration/bradycardia.

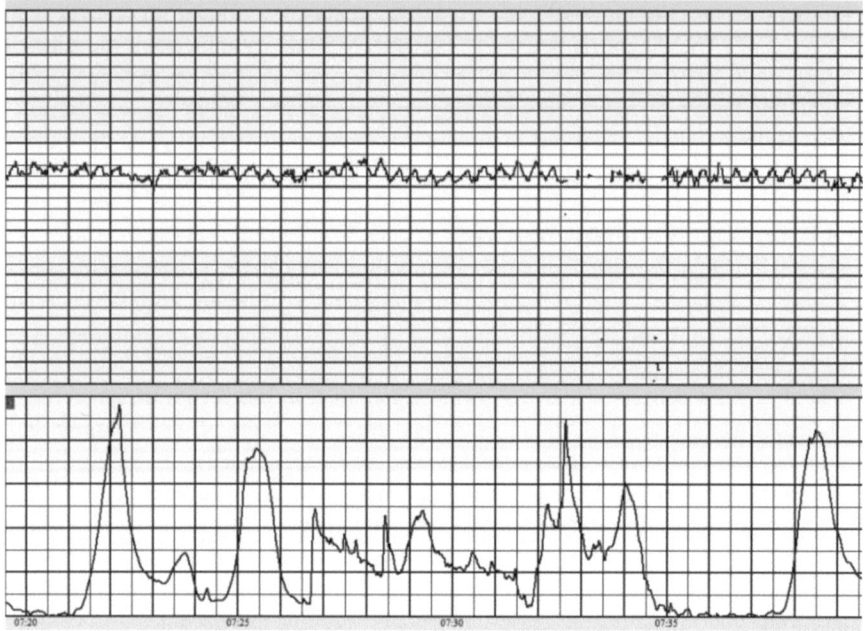

Fig. 2.6 Sinusoidal FHR pattern in fetal-maternal haemorrhage ("paper speed" 1 cm/min)

2.3.5 Specific Mechanical Complications of Labour

Acute fetal hypoxia/acidosis may be caused by specific mechanical complications of labour, associated with umbilical cord compression and/or compression of important fetal blood vessels. The most frequent situations are shoulder dystocia and retention of the after-coming head in vaginal breech delivery. A more detailed description of these situations is provided in Chaps. 3 and 4.

2.4 Clinical Management

The specific management of acute maternal cardiorespiratory arrest, shoulder dystocia and retention of the after-coming head is described in subsequent chapters. The present section is dedicated to management of the remaining causes of acute fetal hypoxia/acidosis.

2.4.1 Immediate Actions in Face of a Prolonged Deceleration

The immediate actions to take when a prolonged deceleration is detected are listed in Table 2.2. The order of these actions may be adapted, if there is a strong suspicion of a specific cause.

2.4 Clinical Management

Table 2.2 Immediate actions in face of a prolonged deceleration

Assure a continuous and good quality FHR signal
Call for help (two midwives, senior obstetrician)
Stop oxytocin, remove prostaglandins. Evaluate contractility (CTG tocograph, palpate uterine fundus to detect tachysystole and/or increased basal tone)
Vaginal examination (to detect umbilical cord prolapse and conditions for instrumental vaginal delivery)
Patient in lateral decubitus (if there are no conditions for immediate delivery)
Evaluate state of consciousness and vital signs (talk to patient, evaluate breathing, radial pulse and blood pressure)

The first consideration should be given to assuring the continuous acquisition of a reliable FHR signal, so that the prolonged deceleration is confirmed, the duration is evaluated, and possible signs of recovery are documented. In addition, the occurrence of reduced variability within the deceleration is very suggestive of fetal hypoxia/acidosis. For all these reasons, continuous CTG should be preferred, if readily available. With external FHR monitoring, it is essential to assure that the fetus rather than the mother is being monitored, so the maternal pulse needs to be simultaneously evaluated to detect coincidences, and frequent repositioning of the Doppler sensor may be required. It is therefore useful to assign one person to assure a continuous good quality FHR signal and to evaluate the maternal pulse intermittently, for an adequate documentation of the situation.

The resolution of most situations of acute fetal hypoxia/acidosis requires a concerted action from a team of healthcare professionals, so therefore help should be promptly summoned, and the presence of at least two midwives and a senior obstetrician assured.

Although many prolonged decelerations revert spontaneously without any intervention, it is sometimes difficult to predict the situations in which this occurs. With the actions described in Table 2.2, all reversible causes of fetal hypoxia/acidosis are quickly identified, and some are immediately corrected. A quick search of the underlying cause is necessary to plan management, as some causes may be quickly reversible (excessive uterine activity, acute maternal hypotension and maternal supine position), while others are irreversible and pose extreme danger to the fetus (major placental abruption, uterine rupture, umbilical cord prolapse). When it is not possible to identify a cause, management should be based mainly on the duration of the deceleration and the evaluation of variability (see below).

Even when there is no apparent tachysystole (see definition above), oxytocin perfusion should be stopped or prostaglandins removed (when possible) to reduce contraction frequency and help recover fetal oxygenation. A vaginal examination is essential to diagnose umbilical cord prolapse and to evaluate the conditions for instrumental vaginal delivery. Even if the patient is in the active second stage of labour, asking the woman to stop pushing and temporary adopting the lateral decubitus position may relieve aorto-caval compression and reduce uterine contraction frequency. In some situations of occult cord compression, it may be the left or the right lateral decubitus that causes the best effect, or alternatively the half-sitting or upright positions.

Table 2.3 Drugs used for acute tocolysis

Salbutamol 125 µg at 25 µ/min IV. One 1 ml vial (0.5 mg/ml) in 100 ml of crystalloid solution, in intravenous perfusion at 300 ml/h for 5 min
Terbutaline 0.25 mg by subcutaneous injection
Atosiban 6.75 mg IV. One 0.9 ml vial (7.5 mg/ml) given by intravenous bolus during 1 min

2.4.2 Uterine Hypercontractility

Uterine hypercontractility occurring when an oxytocin perfusion is in place usually starts to revert 1–3 min after it is stopped, as the half-life of the drug is around 3–6 min. If a faster effect is required or when hypercontractility is spontaneous in nature or prostaglandins cannot be removed, acute tocolysis should be considered (Table 2.3).

Salbutamol and **terbutaline** should not be used in women with coronary artery disease, history of cardiac arrhythmias, high blood pressure, hyperthyroidism or low potassium levels. Their main side effects are tachycardia, tremor and nervousness.

Atosiban has no formal contraindications, but occasional side effects such as headaches, dizziness, vomiting, tachycardia, hypotension and fever have been reported.

Prolonged decelerations should start to revert 1–2 min after acute tocolysis has begun, and waiting for this to occur is the first option when hypercontractility is strongly suspected. During the second stage of labour, instrumental vaginal delivery may be an alternative if there are conditions for a quick and safe procedure. Otherwise, asking the parturient to stop pushing and waiting for reversal of the deceleration is preferable to guarantee the return of adequate fetal oxygenation. It should not be forgotten that uterine hypercontractility may also occur in the initial phases of placental abruption, so the maximum time limits for reversal of a prolonged deceleration should be taken into account (see below).

2.4.3 Sudden Maternal Hypotension

Sudden maternal hypotension secondary to epidural or spinal analgesia is usually quickly reversed by starting or increasing **crystalloid perfusion** and when this is not enough administering **ephedrine** 3–6 mg in intravenous bolus over 5 min. The bolus can be repeated after 5–10 min, until a maximum dose of 10 mg is reached. The drug is contraindicated in patients with cardiac disease, hypertension, hyperthyroidism, phaeocromocytoma and closed angle glaucoma and those who have taken monoamine oxidase inhibitors in the previous 14 days. The following side effects have been reported: paleness, fever, dry mucosae, shortness of breath, chest pain, tachycardia, anxiety, nausea and vomiting, headache, insomnia and mood changes. It can also cause transitory fetal tachycardia.

Administration of colloids is not recommended in these situations, as they can have a negative impact on coagulation, and rare cases of anaphylaxis and acute renal insufficiency have been reported.

Reversal of the FHR deceleration should start very soon after blood pressure begins to normalise, and waiting for this to occur should be the first option unless a very fast and safe instrumental vaginal delivery can be guaranteed. It should not be forgotten that hypotension may also be caused by maternal haemorrhage, as occurs with major placental abruption or uterine rupture, so the maximum time limits for reversal need to be taken into account (see below).

2.4.4 Major Placental Abruption

When major placental abruption is strongly suspected, rapid delivery is required to guarantee the safety of both mother and fetus. Instrumental vaginal delivery may occasionally be possible if there are very favourable conditions, but the majority of cases will present before the active second stage of labour and require emergent caesarean section. The anaesthesiologist and neonatologist should therefore be rapidly summoned and the operating theatre prepared.

Profuse retroplacental haemorrhage and disseminated intravascular coagulation may occur in this situation, so continuous monitoring of maternal vital signs, oxygen saturation and ECG should be started, a vein catheterised with a large bore needle, blood drawn for haemoglobin, coagulation studies and cross-matching and a crystalloid infusion initiated. Blood results need to be monitored regularly in order to identify the first signs of disseminated intravascular coagulation and to anticipate postpartum haemorrhage (see Chap. 7).

If fetal death has occurred and the mother is haemodynamically stable, it is preferable to induce or accelerate labour. In these situations, caesarean section is reserved for absent labour progress, profuse bleeding and/or maternal haemodynamic instability.

As the diagnosis of major placental abruption is not always firmly established before delivery, the maximum time limits for reversal of a prolonged deceleration need to be taken into account (see below).

2.4.5 Uterine Rupture

Uterine rupture requires prompt delivery followed by surgical repair, in order to guarantee the safety of both mother and fetus. Similarly to major placental abruption, when the diagnosis is strongly suspected, continuous monitoring of maternal vital signs, oxygen saturation and ECG should be put in place, a peripheral vein catheterised with a large bore needle, blood drawn for haemoglobin, coagulation studies and cross-matching and a crystalloid infusion initiated. The anaesthesiologist and neonatologist should to be rapidly summoned and the operating theatre prepared.

After confirmation of uterine rupture at laparotomy and delivery of the fetus, surgical correction with a double-layer suture may be technically possible. Several case reports of successful subsequent pregnancies have been described after this type of surgery, usually delivered by elective caesarean section at term. If suturing of the lesion is judged to be impossible, or when it is anticipated to be a lengthy procedure in the context of an unstable patient, peripartum hysterectomy remains the only alternative. Some centres report subtotal hysterectomy to be safer than total hysterectomy in this context, with lower rates of ureteral complications and maternal mortality, but surgical experience should be the determining factor in this choice.

As the diagnosis of uterine rupture cannot always be safely established during labour, particularly when the woman is under epidural or spinal analgesia, the maximum time limits for reversal of a prolonged deceleration need to be taken into account (see below).

2.4.6 Umbilical Cord Prolapse

When umbilical cord prolapse occurs in the absence of continuous CTG monitoring, cord pulsatility should be evaluated, and if doubt remains as to the occurrence of blood flow, heart movements should be quickly confirmed on ultrasound. A few cases of fetal survival have been reported when rapid action is taken in spite of an apparently non-pulsatile cord. An exteriorised umbilical loop requires as little manipulation as possible to avoid vascular spasm.

If the fetus is alive and the gestational age is viable, immediate measures should be taken to reduce cord compression and quickly deliver the fetus, usually by caesarean section. Cord prolapse is very rare during the second stage of labour with the head fully engaged, so instrumental vaginal delivery is usually not an option. The patient should be rapidly placed in a **head-down position** and the **presenting part raised** by a hand inside the vagina, measures that are maintained until delivery. An anaesthesiologist and a neonatologist need to be rapidly summoned, the operating theatre prepared and the patient transported there as quickly as possible.

When immediate caesarean delivery is not possible (i.e. when prolapse occurs in a health facility that does not have an operating theatre), acute tocolysis should be started (Table 2.3), the bladder catheterised and 500–750 ml of saline solution instilled via the catheter in order to maintain the presenting part elevated. Continuous monitoring by CTG or handheld Doppler is then maintained during patient transport, until a caesarean section is performed.

Currently, there is insufficient evidence on the safety of alternative treatments for umbilical cord prolapse, such as digital reduction of the prolapsed cord followed by expectant management, although there are a few reported cases of success in the scientific literature.

2.4.7 Maximum Time Limits for Reversal of a Prolonged Deceleration

Frequently, the underlying cause of a prolonged deceleration is not clear, and no safe judgement can be made as to its reversible or irreversible nature, nor of the probability of recurrence when contractility is resumed. Abundant vaginal bleeding is highly suggestive of an irreversible cause (placental abruption, uterine rupture, ruptured vasa praevia) and should prompt immediate delivery. The appearance of a sinusoidal pattern is also very suggestive of fetal haemorrhage (fetal-maternal haemorrhage or ruptured vasa praevia) and should also motivate rapid delivery.

Whatever the cause of fetal hypoxia/acidosis, maximum time limits for a prolonged deceleration need to be established in order to guarantee the absence of permanent injury to the fetus.

Particular care is recommended when prolonged decelerations exceed **5 min** and there is no tendency to recover, especially when there is reduced variability within the deceleration. The healthcare team should start preparing all the requirements needed for a rapid caesarean section or instrumental vaginal delivery. The latter should only be considered if a quick and safe procedure can be guaranteed; otherwise the operating theatre team should be prepared for an emergent caesarean section. The anaesthesiologist and neonatologist should be rapidly summoned. The final decision to intervene depends on local conditions, such as distance to the operating theatre and the team's proficiency with the surgery, as well as on additional clinical information (normal or growth-retarded fetus, previous CTG changes, appearance of vaginal bleeding or other symptoms suggesting an irreversible cause). With an adequately grown and previously well-oxygenated fetus at term, this decision should rarely go beyond **7–8 min**. The whole team must be aware of the urgency of the situation, and the fetus needs to be **delivered within 3–4 min**, so that the total duration of the hypoxic insult does not exceed 12 min.

2.5 Clinical Records and Litigation Issues

The complications of intrapartum fetal hypoxia/acidosis constitute major causes of litigation in high- and medium-resource countries. Extreme care needs therefore to be taken with clinical records, so that it is clear which healthcare professionals were called, at what time they were called, when did they arrive, as well as who took which decisions, and who performed which procedures.

It is also very important to document umbilical artery blood pH and base deficit (or alternatively lactate) in all situations where there has been an obstetric intervention for suspected fetal hypoxia/acidosis and when Apgar scores are low. This information is important to increase the team's knowledge with management of these situations, and it also allows a clarification of many causes of neonatal encephalopathy, perinatal mortality and cerebral palsy. A large number of these complications are not due to intrapartum hypoxia/acidosis, and they can be ruled out with this information.

During caesarean section, it is important to look for causes of acute fetal hypoxia/acidosis, as some may only be revealed at this time. Major placental abruption may result in the formation of a retroplacental haematoma and/or a Couvelaire uterus, and histological examination of the placenta will confirm the diagnosis. Tight nuchal chords, true cord knots, low-lying cord loops and ruptured umbilical/placental vessels can usually be detected during caesarean section or at subsequent inspection of the placenta and membranes. Fetal haemorrhage requires the documentation of newborn anaemia, and fetal-maternal haemorrhage can be detected by the Kleihauer-Betke test or flow cytometry.

A clear explanation of the situation to the parents, during and shortly after it has occurred, frequently removes main of the misunderstandings and uncertainties that lead to litigation. The obstetric team also needs to remain informed of the health status of the newborn, so that all information conveyed to the mother and family is coherent and adapted to this evolution.

MANAGEMENT OF A PROLONGED FHR DECELERATION

Initial measures	Continuous CTG, evaluate maternal pulse	☐
	Evaluate duration of deceleration and variability	☐
	Call for help (two midwives, senior obstetrician)	☐
	Stop oxytocin, prostaglandins. Evaluate contractility	☐
	Vaginal examination	☐
	Patient in lateral decubitus	☐
	Evaluate state of consciousness and vital signs	☐
1. Hypercontractility	Acute tocolysis if needed	☐
2. Maternal hypotension	Start/increase crystalloid perfusion	☐
	Ephedrin in intravenous bolus	☐

3. Suspected major placental abruption or uterine rupture

	Continuous BP, HR, O_2 sat, ECG	☐
	Venous catheterisation with large bore catheter	☐
	Blood samples (Hb, coagulation, cross-matching)	☐
	Crystalloid perfusion	☐
	Rapid cesarean section /laparotomy	☐
3. Umbilical cord prolapse	Head-down position	☐
	Manual elevation of the presenting part	☐
	Emergent cesarean section	☐

5. Acute maternal cardio-repiratory disorder (see chapter 7)

6. Specific mechanical complications of labour (see following chapters)

7. General rules (adequately-grown, previously well-oxygenated term fetuses)

Deceleration 5-6 minutes	Call anesthesiologist and neonatologist	☐
	Prepare operating theatre or instrumental delivery	☐
Deceleration 7-8 minutes	Rapid c-section or instrumental vaginal delivery	☐
Documentation	Umbilical blood sampling and analysis	☐
	Register all occurrences	☐

Suggested Reading

American College of Obstetricians and Gynecologists (1993) Fetal and neonatal neurologic injury (technical bulletin number 163). Int J Gynecol Obstet 41:97–101

American College of Obstetricians and Gynecologists (1996) Umbilical artery blood acid-base analysis (technical bulletin). Int J Gynecol Obstet 52:305–310

Ayres-de-Campos D, Arulkumaran S, for the FIGO Intrapartum Fetal Monitoring Expert Consensus Panel (2015a) FIGO consensus guidelines on intrapartum fetal monitoring: physiology of fetal oxygenation and the main goals of intrapartum fetal monitoring. Int J Gynecol Obstet 131:5–8

Ayres-de-Campos D, Spong CY, Chandraharan E, for the FIGO Intrapartum Fetal Monitoring Expert Consensus Panel (2015b) FIGO consensus guidelines on intrapartum fetal monitoring: cardiotocography. Int J Gynecol Obstet 131:13–24

Doria V, Papageorghiou A, Gustafsson A, Ugwumadu A, Farrer K, Arulkumaran S (2007) Review of the first 1502 cases of ECG-ST waveform analysis during labour in a teaching hospital. BJOG 114:1202–1207

Giacoia GP (1997) Severe fetomaternal hemorrhage: a review. Obstet Gynecol Surv 52(6):372–380

Giwa-Osagie OF, Uguru V, Akinla O (1983) Mortality and morbidity of emergency obstetric hysterectomy. Obstet Gynecol 4:94–96

Goswami K (2007) Umbilical cord prolapse. In: Grady K, Howell C, Cox C (eds) Managing obstetric emergencies and trauma. The MOET course manual, 2nd edn. RCOG Press, London

Hofmeyr G, Cyna A, Middleton P (2004) Prophylactic intravenous preloading for regional analgesia in labour. Cochrane Database Syst Rev (4):CD000175

Katz VL, Dotters DJ, Droegemueller W (1986) Perimortem cesarean delivery. Obstet Gynecol 68:571–576

Lin MG (2006) Umbilical cord prolapse. Obstet Gynecol Surv 61:269–277

Low JA, Lindsay BG, Derrick EJ (1997) Threshold of metabolic acidosis associated with newborn complications. Am J Obstet Gynecol 177:1391–1394

MacLennan A for the International Cerebral Palsy Task Force (1999) A template for defining a causal relation between acute intrapartum events and cerebral palsy: international consensus statement. BMJ 319:1054–1059

Morgan JL, Casey BM, Bloom SL, McIntire DD, Leveno KJ (2015) Metabolic acidemia in live births at 35 weeks of gestation or greater. Obstet Gynecol 126(2):279–283

National Collaborating Centre for Women's and Children's Health (2007) Intrapartum care: care of healthy women and their babies during childbirth (clinical guideline). RCOG Press, London

Norén H, Carlsson A (2010) Reduced prevalence of metabolic acidosis at birth: an analysis of established STAN usage in the total population of deliveries in a Swedish district hospital. Am J Obstet Gynecol 202(6):546e.1–546e.7

Rasmussen S, Irgens LM, Bergsjo P, Dalaker K (1996) The occurrence of placental abruption in Norway 1967-1991. Acta Obstet Gynecol Scand 75:222–228

Royal College of Obstetricians and Gynaecologists (2011) Placenta praevia, placenta praevia accrete and vasa praevia: diagnosis and mangament (Green-top guideline no. 28). RCOG Press, London

Rubod C, Deruelle P, Le Goueff F, Tunez V, Fournier M, Subtil D (2007) Long-term prognosis for infants after massive fetomaternal hemorrhage. Obstet Gynecol 110(2 Pt 1):256–260

Ruth VJ, Raivio KO (1988) Perinatal brain damage: predictive value of metabolic acidosis and the Apgar score. BMJ 297:24–27

van de Riet JE, Vandenbussche FPHA, Le Cessie S, Keirse MJNC (1999) Newborn assessment and long-term adverse outcome: a systematic review. Am J Obstet Gynecol 180:1024–1029

World Health Organization, UNFPA, UNICEF, World Bank (2003) Managing complications in pregnancy and childbirth. A guide for midwives and doctors. Prolapsed cord. WHO Press, Geneva. S-97–98. [www.who.int/reproductive-health/impac/index.html]

Shoulder Dystocia 3

3.1 Definition, Incidence and Main Risk Factors

The term shoulder dystocia describes a series of difficulties encountered with release of the fetal shoulders in cephalic deliveries and more objectively the need to use additional manoeuvres when axial traction on the fetal head has failed. An overall incidence between 0.58 and 0.70 % of vaginal deliveries is reported in the largest observational studies.

The **main mechanism** behind the occurrence of shoulder dystocia is the retention of the anterior shoulder behind the pubic symphysis, while the posterior shoulder is usually located in the maternal pelvis (Fig. 3.1). In rare situations, both shoulders are retained above the pelvic brim.

The main **risk factors** for shoulder dystocia are listed in Table 3.1. **Previous shoulder dystocia** stands out as a major risk factor for recurrence, and it is reported to be

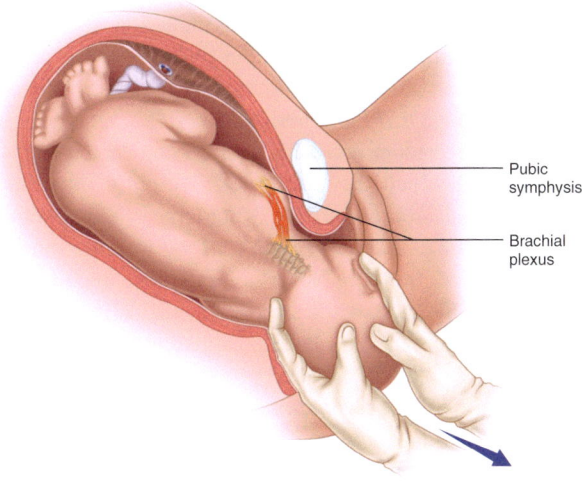

Fig. 3.1 The main mechanism behind the occurrence of shoulder dystocia – retention of the anterior fetal shoulder above the pubic symphysis

© Springer International Publishing Switzerland 2017
D. Ayres-de-Campos, *Obstetric Emergencies*,
DOI 10.1007/978-3-319-41656-4_3

Table 3.1 Main risk factors for shoulder dystocia

Previous shoulder dystocia
Fetal macrosomia and its associated risk factors
Pre-existing or gestational diabetes
Maternal obesity
Excessive weight gain during pregnancy
Post-term pregnancy
Slow progress of labour
Prolonged first and/or second stage
Need for labour acceleration
Instrumental vaginal delivery

10-times higher than in the general population, for an overall incidence of 1–25 %. The anatomical characteristics of the maternal pelvis that predispose to shoulder dystocia and may cause it to be recurrent in nature are poorly understood. When additional risk factors are present, such as maternal diabetes or suspected fetal macrosomia or when previous fetal injury occurred in association with shoulder dystocia, serious consideration should be given to elective caesarean delivery, and this option should be discussed with the mother. In the remaining situations, management remains controversial.

Another major risk factor is **fetal macrosomia**, and when coexistent with poorly controlled **maternal diabetes**, an additional 2–4-fold risk is present, posed by the increased diameter of the fetal shoulders.

With isolated macrosomia, there is recent evidence from a randomised controlled trial that fetuses whose estimated weight is above the 95th percentile close to term benefit from induction of labour at 37–38 weeks, as it reduces the risk of shoulder dystocia by about 70 % and also slightly increases the number of vaginal deliveries. An estimated fetal weight above 5000 g is considered in many guidelines to be an indication for elective caesarean section, and others include this recommendation for estimated weights above 4500 g.

With maternal diabetes, labour induction at 38–39 weeks has been shown to decrease the incidence of shoulder dystocia and is recommended in several guidelines. Some institutions recommend elective caesarean section when estimated fetal weight is above 4250 g or above 4500 g.

The above recommendations have been criticised for the limited strength of the evidence on which they are based. Weight estimation by ultrasound has a well-demonstrated inherent error, particularly in macrosomic fetuses. One should also not forget that caesarean section for fetal weights above 4500 g is associated with a 2.5 % risk of trauma. Nevertheless, these recommendations remain important sources of guidance, while stronger evidence is awaited.

Risk factors that only become apparent during labour are more difficult to integrate into the clinical decision process. In spite of significant associations existing between all of these risk factors and shoulder dystocia, none of them are sufficiently discriminative to allow an accurate prediction. The majority of cases of shoulder dystocia occur in pregnancies that have no risk factors, and when one is present, the majority of cases do not develop this complication. There is therefore wide agreement within the medical community that shoulder dystocia is generally an

unpredictable situation. Nevertheless, identification of risk factors is useful for anticipating of the situation, so that an experienced team can be on hand at the time of delivery.

3.2 Complications

The most frequent complication of shoulder dystocia is **brachial plexus injury**, of which Erb's palsy is the usual presentation. The latter manifests by a characteristic position of the affected arm that hangs by the side of the body and is rotated medially. The forearm is usually extended and pronate (Fig. 3.2). It affects about 0.15 % of all births, and in some countries, the incidence appears to be decreasing. Older studies report brachial plexus injury to occur in 2–16 % of shoulder dystocias, but recent data from centres performing regular staff training refer that this can be reduced to about 1.3 %. Brachial plexus injury appears to be related mainly to the traction force applied on the fetal head. Improved awareness of the fact and simulation-based training of the force that can be safely applied to the fetal head may be responsible for the decreasing incidence of this complication.

The underlying cause for injury is believed to be exaggerated mechanical distention of the brachial nerve, but the mechanism is incompletely understood, as it may also affect the posterior arm, and cases have been reported to occur in elective

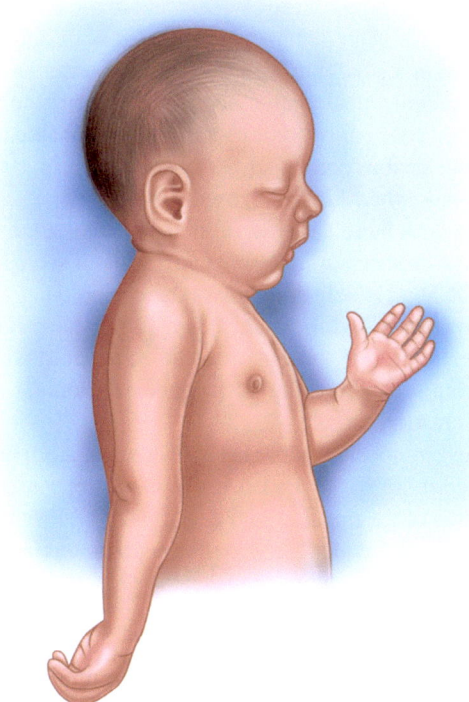

Fig. 3.2 Newborn with a right arm position typical of Erb's paralysis

caesarean section and vaginal delivery without shoulder dystocia. In 24–53 % of brachial plexus injuries, no documentation of shoulder dystocia was found, and 4–12 % occurred after caesarean section, so it is possible that they are also caused by abnormal intrauterine fetal positions.

Of all brachial plexus injuries diagnosed at birth, the majority disappear after treatment, and only 10–23 % remain after 12 months. In the majority of cases of residual paralysis, some degree of recovery is achievable after surgery.

Shoulder dystocia is also a cause of **perinatal mortality**, although the incidence appears to have decreased in the last decades. Confidential enquiries carried out in the United Kingdom indicate that it may be responsible for about 8 % of intrapartum fetal deaths. The main cause of perinatal death is **acute fetal hypoxia/acidosis** (see Chap. 2).

There is uncertainty about how many minutes may elapse before the fetus is at risk of injury from acute hypoxia/acidosis. The phenomenon is probably faster when there are nuchal cords and when cord clamping takes place before the shoulders are released. Five such cases with resolution taking 3–7 min were reported in association with cerebral palsy, but it is uncertain whether intrapartum hypoxia/acidosis was already present before delivery of the head. Sustained cord occlusion is likely to occur in these situations, and therefore umbilical blood gas values may not translate the severity of hypoxia/acidosis. Hypoxic-ischaemic encephalopathy has been documented in cases with only moderate acidaemia on cord gas analysis.

Compression of fetal neck vessels may also play an important part in the pathophysiological mechanism, and it may be the main cause of cerebral injury when no nuchal cords are present. Again, umbilical blood gas values may not translate the severity of hypoxia/acidosis occurring in the brain, and hypoxic-ischaemic encephalopathy has been documented in cases with only moderate acidemia on cord gas analysis. In a small but well-documented observational study, no cases of hypoxic-ischaemic encephalopathy were found when resolution took less than 5 min, and only mild cases of hypoxic-ischaemic encephalopathy were reported when it lasted 5–9 min. Serious complications of hypoxia/acidosis were only described in one case where more than 12 min elapsed.

Although there are no certainties as to the time that may elapse before the fetus is at risk of injury from hypoxia/acidosis, it seems wise not to clamp nuchal cords after the head is delivered unless there is no other alternative and to attempt resolution preferably within 5 min. When 12 min have elapsed, fetal prognosis is likely to be poor. Different timings must be considered when fetal oxygenation is already compromised before the occurrence of shoulder dystocia or when there is fetal growth restriction.

Rarer complications of shoulder dystocia are **fractures of clavicle and humerus**, the majority of which are iatrogenic in nature, consequent to the manoeuvres used for resolution of the situation, and they usually heal without sequelae after immobilisation.

The most frequent maternal complications are **vaginal and perineal lacerations**, and some studies report anal sphincter lacerations to occur in about 4 % of shoulder dystocia cases.

Postpartum haemorrhage affects about 11 % of cases and can be caused by birth canal lacerations and more frequently by uterine atony. Rare cases of uterine rupture, bladder rupture, dehiscence of the pubic symphysis and sacroiliac joint dislocation have also been described.

3.3 Diagnosis

The most common definition of shoulder dystocia is the **need to use additional manoeuvres** to release the fetal shoulders, after the usual axial traction on the head has failed. However, it is important to add that traction should be continuous and that it should not exceed a maximum force of 100 Newtons. No more than two or three tractions should be applied before the diagnosis is established.

Other criteria have been proposed for the definition of shoulder dystocia, based on the time interval between delivery of the fetal head and release of the shoulders, and they consider cut-offs of 1 or 2 min. However, accurate measurement of these intervals may not be practicable in many hospitals.

3.4 Clinical Management

3.4.1 Anticipating the Situation

When risk factors are identified (Table 3.2) or when premonitory signs are detected, steps should be taken to summon an experienced healthcare team, in case shoulder dystocia occurs. Moving the mother closer to the end of the bed or removing the lower part of the bed may also be useful, to improve access to the fetal head.

The most important premonitory signs are a marked descent of the fetal head during pushing followed by an abnormal rise in between contractions and the turtle sign, a situation where there is incomplete expulsion of the fetal head, so that the fetal mandible and occiput remain depressing the maternal perineum (Fig. 3.3).

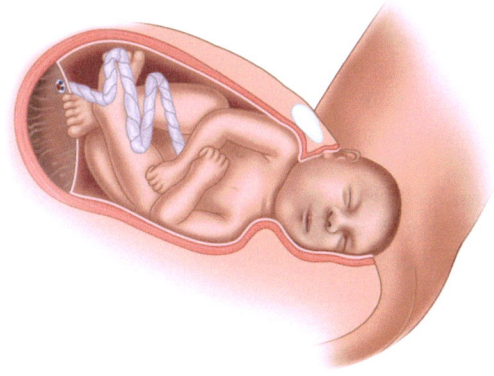

Fig. 3.3 Turtle sign, with the lower structures of the fetal head depressing the maternal perineum

3.4.2 Clearly Verbalising the Diagnosis

In these situations, it is important to convey the diagnosis to all healthcare professionals present in the room, so that the team may act accordingly, and therefore it needs to be clearly verbalised, without unnecessarily alarming the labouring woman and her companion.

3.4.3 Avoiding Manoeuvres That Increase the Risk of Fetal Injury

The manoeuvres most frequently associated with brachial plexus injury are excessive traction on the fetal head, non-axial traction and forced rotation. Fundal pressure should also be avoided, as it only serves to push the anterior shoulder against the pubic symphysis. Maternal pushing has a similar effect, so the mother should be asked to stop this.

3.4.4 Asking for Help

Management of shoulder dystocia requires a concerted effort from the healthcare team, so one of the first measures should be to summon at least two midwives and a senior obstetrician. In addition, a neonatologist and an anaesthetist should be called, the first one because neonatal resuscitation is likely to be required and the second because uterine relaxation is sometimes needed for the internal manoeuvres (see below).

3.4.5 External Manoeuvres

External manoeuvres resolve the vast majority of shoulder dystocia cases and should be attempted first:

McRobert's Manoeuvre Hyperflexion of the mother's thighs against her abdomen – this manoeuvre is performed by two assistants, one on each side of the mother, each holding one leg and forcibly flexing and abducting the thighs against the lateral part of the abdomen (Fig. 3.4). After this is accomplished, gentle and continuous axial traction on the fetal head is reattempted. With this manoeuvre, the lumbosacral angle is straightened, and the pubic symphysis is moved anterosuperiorly, thus helping the anterior shoulder to slip under the pubic bone.

Suprapubic Pressure This is usually performed by one of the assistants executing the McRobert's manoeuvre (Fig. 3.4), with a closed hand applying firm and sustained pressure above the pubic symphysis. After this is in place, gentle and continuous axial traction on the fetal head is reattempted. The applied pressure helps the anterior shoulder to slip under the pubic bone. As an alternative, some authors advocate the use of strong and intermittent suprapubic pressure (Rubin I manoeuvre), but there is no evidence on comparative efficacies.

Fig. 3.4 McRobert's manoeuvre performed together with suprapubic pressure

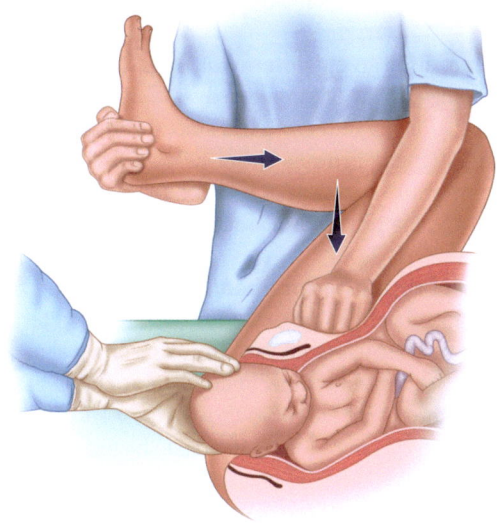

Fig. 3.5 Rotation of the anterior shoulder

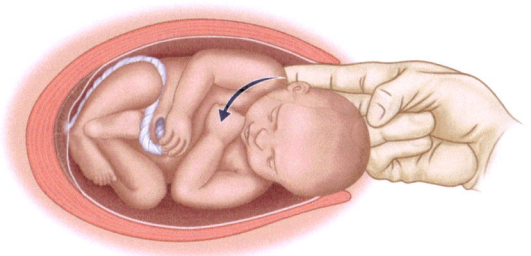

3.4.6 Internal Manoeuvres

Internal manoeuvres should be performed by the most experienced healthcare professional available, while two assistants maintain the McRobert's manoeuvre. There is no clear evidence on which order the internal manoeuvres should be performed, so this depends more on the experience of the executor and the accessibility of the different fetal structures. Nevertheless, the order presented here reflects the logical sequence of increasing difficulty.

Rotation of the Anterior Shoulder (Rubin II manoeuvre) – One or two fingers are introduced behind the anterior shoulder, and apply continuous and firm pressure to slowly rotate it in the direction of the fetal thorax (Fig. 3.5). At the same time, one of the assistants performing the McRobert's manoeuvre applies suprapubic pressure laterally, to help rotate the anterior shoulder in the same direction. Sometimes it is possible to use one finger of the contralateral hand to simultaneously rotate the posterior shoulder towards the fetal back. The shoulders should be rotated between 45° and 90°, after which axial traction is reapplied on the fetal head.

The need for an **episiotomy** or for extension of an existing one is controversial in the management of shoulder dystocia. In the past, it was part of many management guidelines, but its role has since been questioned and it has ceased to be used routinely in many centres. Nevertheless, it may be useful in situations where access to the posterior shoulder for rotation or extraction of the posterior arm is made difficult by the maternal perineum.

Rotation of the Posterior Shoulder (Woods corkscrew manoeuvre) – Two fingers are introduced behind the posterior shoulder or alternatively the whole hand is introduced around it, to rotate the shoulder slowly but firmly towards the fetal thorax (Fig. 3.6). At the same time, lateral suprapubic pressure is applied by an assistant to rotate the anterior shoulder in the direction of the fetal back. Sometimes, one finger of the executer's contralateral hand can be used simultaneously, to rotate the anterior shoulder towards the fetal back. Again the rotation should be of 45–90° after which axial traction is reapplied on the fetal head.

Extraction of the Posterior Arm The whole hand is introduced in the vagina around the posterior shoulder, following the fetal arm until the elbow. Using the tips of the fingers, the forearm is flexed and the pulse grabbed to extract the hand, followed by the arm, along the fetal body and head (Fig. 3.7). Once extracted, the posterior arm is used as a lever to rotate the posterior shoulder 45–90° in the direction of the thorax, thus releasing the anterior shoulder. In small observational studies, a 2–13 % rate of humeral fractures was reported with this manoeuvre, but this could have been due to the relative inexperience of the executors.

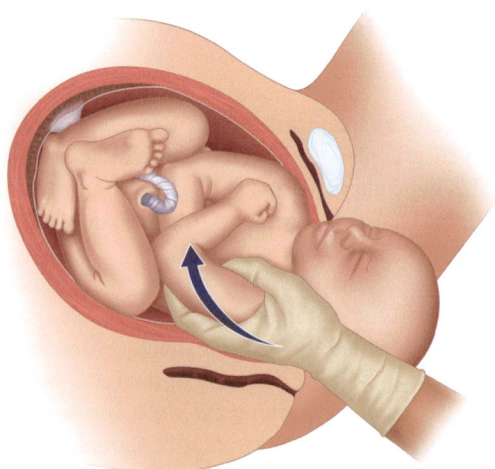

Fig. 3.6 Rotation of the posterior shoulder

3.4 Clinical Management

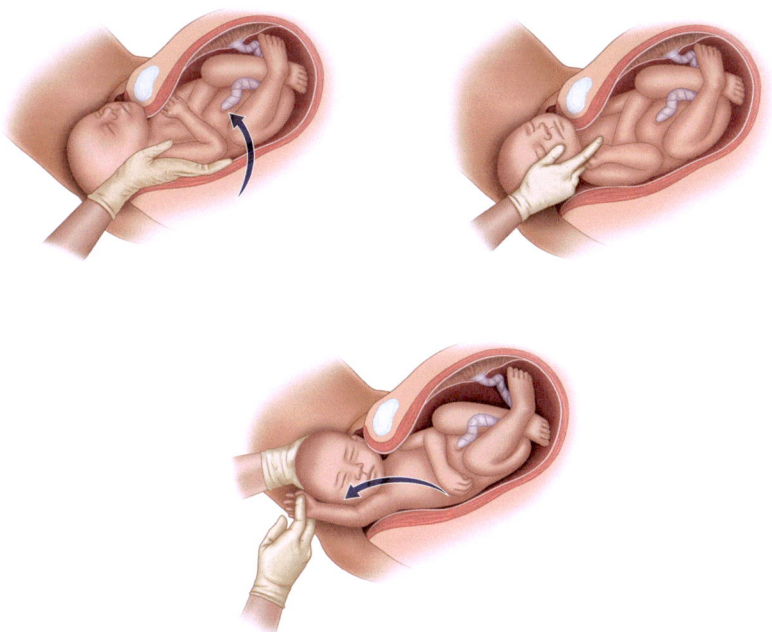

Fig. 3.7 Extraction of the posterior arm

Table 3.2 Medications used for uterine relaxation

Nitroglicerin in slow intravenous bolus (50–100 µg IV slowly). One 5 ml vial (5 mg/ml) in 500 ml of saline. Slow intravenous injection of 1–2 ml (50–100 µg) with continuous blood pressure monitoring
Salbutamol in intravenous perfusion (125 µg at 25 µ/min). One vial of 1 ml (0.5 mg/ml) in 100 ml of saline in intravenous perfusion at 300 ml/h during 5 min

Uterine relaxation is usually not required for executing the internal manoeuvres, but sometimes pressure inside the uterine cavity prevents mobilisation of the shoulders or extraction of the posterior arm. Uterine relaxants may be useful in these situations (Table 3.2).

3.4.7 All-Fours Manoeuvre (Gaskin's Manoeuvre)

This manoeuvre consists of placing the labouring woman on her hands and knees and applying continuous and gentle axial traction on the fetal head, to release what was previously the posterior shoulder (Fig. 3.8). Its place in the shoulder dystocia management protocol is currently unclear, particularly in hospital environments. It is mostly used in community settings when only one birth attendant is present and where an 83 % success rate has been reported. In hospital settings, it may be attempted before the exceptional manoeuvres described below are considered.

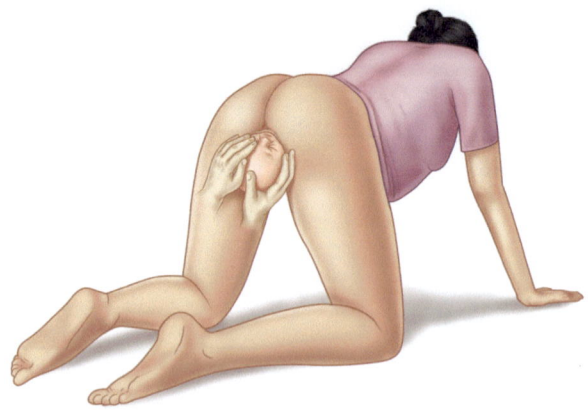

Fig. 3.8 All-fours manoeuvre with axial traction being applied on the fetal head

3.4.8 Exceptional Manoeuvres

Situations of shoulder dystocia that are not resolved with the manoeuvres described above are very rare, and by the time exceptional manoeuvres are considered, fetal prognosis may already be poor. Nevertheless, the problem still requires resolution. The patient needs to be **transferred to the operating theatre**, because general anaesthesia with halogenated agents is required for the Zavanelli manoeuvre. Some consider a final repetition of the internal manoeuvres in the operating theatre under general anaesthesia, because of the more effective uterine relaxation.

Zavanelli's Manoeuvre (Cephalic replacement followed by caesarean section) – this manoeuvre was described for the first time in 1978, and it is performed in the operating theatre under general anaesthesia with halogenated agents. The manoeuvre starts with slow rotation of the fetal head to an occiput-anterior position, followed by flexion of the fetal neck and application of firm and continuous pressure for the reintroduction of the fetal head in the maternal pelvis (Fig. 3.9). An immediate caesarean section follows. A small number of case series are reported in the literature with varying success rates and usually low maternal morbidity, but uterine rupture and subsequent need for hysterectomy have also been described. When fetal prognosis is reserved, maternal morbidity becomes the main priority, and this is probably the less traumatic alternative for her.

Symphysiotomy This technique has been described for the resolution of obstructed labour since the nineteenth century, but its current use in high-resource countries is limited to cases of shoulder dystocia and retention of the after-coming head (see Chap. 4). Symphysiotomy is associated with important maternal morbidity, so it should probably be the last option when fetal prognosis is poor. The procedure can be performed under regional, general and local anaesthesia with opiate sedation. It should be preceded by antibiotic prophylaxis, bladder catheterisation, shaving and disinfection of the pubic area. Before incision, two assistants hold the mother's legs 60–80° apart, after removing them from the bed stirrups. This avoids sudden leg abduction when the symphysis is opened, which can cause urethral injury. With a hand introduced in the vagina to push the urethra aside, a transabdominal vertical incision is performed with a long scalpel between the lower two-thirds and the upper

Fig. 3.9 Zavanelli's manoeuvre

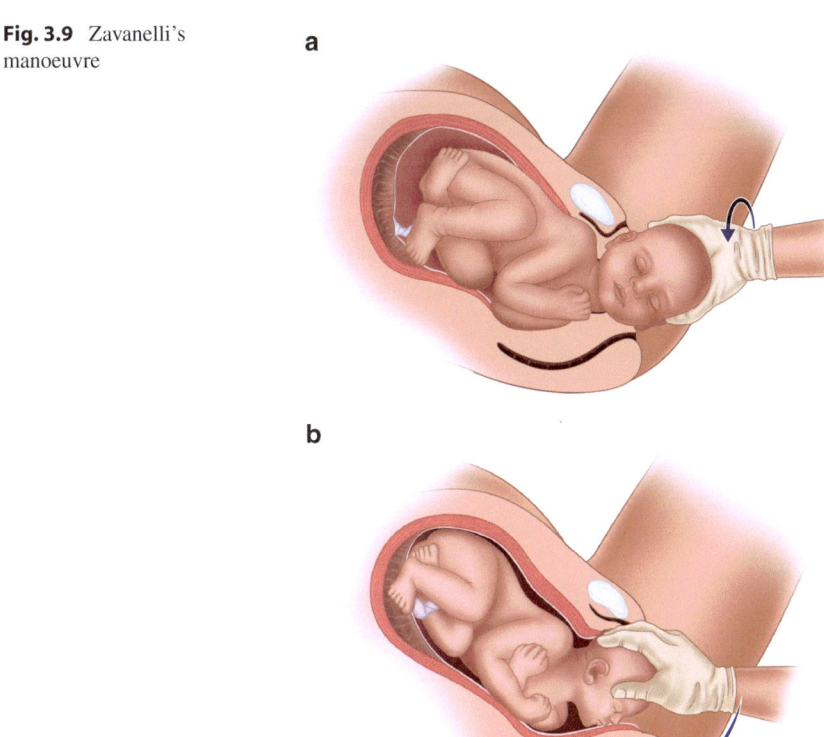

third of the pubic symphysis (Fig. 3.10). Pushing the handle upwards will open the lower two-thirds. The scalpel is then reintroduced into the incision with the blade facing upwards and the handle pushed downwards to open the remaining upper third. It is usually possible to separate the pubic bones by about 2–3 cm, and this allows the shoulders to be released. After closing the abdominal skin, the maternal pelvis is bound with an orthopaedic strap, and bladder catheterisation is maintained for 48 h.

In the absence of complications, the patient is maintained in lateral decubitus for two days, and assisted walking starts on the third. Among the reported complications are para-urethral lacerations, vulval oedema and skin incision haematomas. Difficulties in mobilisation may persist for several months in 1–2 % of cases.

3.5 Clinical Records and Litigation Issues

A comprehensive understanding of the mechanism and consequences of shoulder dystocia is not frequent in expecting mothers nor is the notion that the situation is usually unpredictable. Litigation continues to be common in cases of adverse outcome, so strict adherence to management algorithms, together with carefully written clinical records is required. It is important to document the time at which the head and the

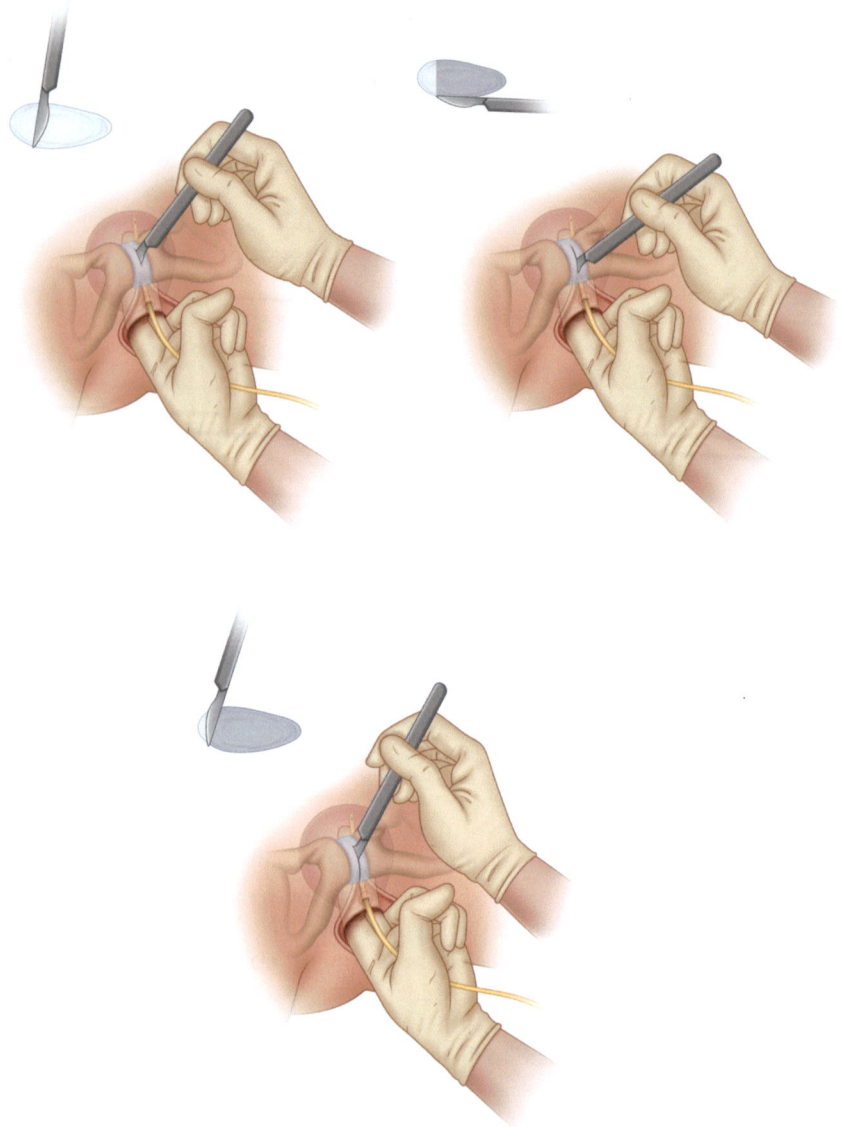

Fig. 3.10 The main steps of symphysiotomy

shoulders were released, which fetal shoulder was in the anterior position, who were the healthcare professionals summoned, when they were called and when they arrived, which manoeuvres were performed, when and by whom. It is usually convenient to have a structured pro forma for registering the management of shoulder dystocia, either in paper or in an electronic format, so that all these details are not forgotten.

Complications secondary to fetal hypoxia/acidosis are the most serious, so it is important to document umbilical blood gas values and Apgar scores at birth.

Finally, a clear and frank explanation of the occurrence to the parents frequently removes much of the suspicion, disinformation and misunderstanding that lead to litigation. The healthcare team needs to remain informed of the health status of the newborn, so that conveyed information is adapted to this evolution.

MANAGEMENT OF SHOULDER DYSTOCIA

Diagnosis	Continuous gentle axial traction on the head	☐
	Clear verbalisation of the diagnosis	☐
Avoid fetal injury	Stop maternal pushing	☐
	Avoid fundal pressure	☐
	Avoid non-axial traction and rotation of the fetal head	☐
Ask for help	At least two midwives	☐
	Senior obstetrician	☐
	Neonatologist	☐
	Anesthetist	☐
External maneuvers	McRobert's maneuver	☐
	Suprapubic pressure	☐
Internal maneuvers	Rotation of the anterior shoulder (Rubin II)	☐
	Episiotomy or extension (if needed)	☐
	Rotation of the posterior shoulder (Woods)	☐
	Extraction of the posterior arm	☐
	Uterine relaxation (if needed)	☐
	Consider Gaskin's Exceptional maneuvers	☐
Exceptional maneuvers	Transport to the operating theatre	☐
	General anesthesia with halogenated agents	☐
	Consider repetition of the internal maneuvers	☐
	Zavanelli's maneuver	☐
	Symphyisiotomy	☐
Documentation	Cord blood sampling	☐
	People called, at what time, and when they arrived	☐
	Maneuvers performed, when and by whom	☐

Suggested Reading

Allan RH, Bankoski BR, Butzin CA, Nagey DA (1994) Comparing clinician-applied loads for routine, difficult and shoulder dystocia deliveries. Am J Obstet Gynecol 171:1621–1627

Boulvain M, Senat MV, Perrotin F, Winer N, Beucher G, Subtil D, Bretelle F, Azria E, Hejaiej D, Vendittelli F, Capelle M, Langer B, Matis R, Connan L, Gillard P, Kirkpatrick C, Ceysens G,

Faron G, Irion O, Rozenberg P, Groupe de Recherche en Obstétrique et Gynécologie (GROG) (2015) Induction of labour versus expectant management for large-for-date fetuses: a randomised controlled trial. Lancet 385(9987):2600–2605

Boulvain M, Stan C, Irion O (2001) Elective delivery in diabetic pregnant women. Cochrane Database Syst Rev (2):CD001997

Bruner JP, Drummond SB, Meenan AL, Gaskin IM (1998) All-fours maneuver for reducing shoulder dystocia during labor. J Reprod Med 43:439–443

Buhimschi CS, Buhimschi IA, Malinow A, Weiner CP (2001) Use of McRoberts' position during delivery and increase in pushing efficiency. Lancet 358:470–471

Chauhan SP, Blackwell SB, Ananth CV (2014) Neonatal brachial plexus palsy: incidence, prevalence, and temporal trends. Semin Perinatol 38(4):210–218

Crofts JF, Lenguerrand E, Bentham GL, Tawfik S, Claireaux HA, Odd D, Fox R, Draycott TJ (2016) Prevention of brachial plexus injury-12 years of shoulder dystocia training: an interrupted time-series study. BJOG 123(1):111–118

Evans-Jones G, Kay SP, Weindling AM, Cranny G, Ward A, Bradshaw A, Hernon C (2003) Congenital brachial plexus injury: incidence, causes and outcome in the UK and Republic of Ireland. Arch Dis Child Fetal Neonatal Ed 88:F185–F189

Gherman RB, Ouzounian JG, Satin AJ, Goodwin TM, Phelan JP (2003) A comparison of shoulder dystocia-associated transient and permanent brachial plexus palsies. Obstet Gynecol 102:544–548

Hinshaw K (2003) Shoulder dystocia. In: Johanson R, Cox C, Grady K, Howell C (eds) Managing obstetric emergencies and trauma: the MOET course manual. RCOG Press, London, pp 165–174

Hope P, Breslin S, Lamont L, Lucas A, Martin D, Moore I, Pearson J, Saunders D, Settatree R (1998) Fatal shoulder dystocia: a review of 56 cases reported to the Confidential Enquiry into Stillbirths and Deaths in Infancy. Br J Obstet Gynaecol 105:1256–1261

Iffy L, Varadi V (1994) Cerebral palsy following cutting of the nuchal cord before delivery. Med Law 13(3–4):323–330

Irion O, Boulvain M (2000) Induction of labour for suspected fetal macrosomia. Cochrane Database Syst Rev (2):CD000938

Leung T, Stuart O, Sahota D, Suen S, Lau T, Lao T (2011) Head-to-body delivery interval and risk of fetal acidosis and hypoxic ischaemic encephalopathy in shoulder dystocia: a retrospective review. BJOG 118:474–479

Naef RW 3rd, Morrison JC (1994) Guidelines for management of shoulder dystocia. J Perinatol 14:435–441

O'Leary J (1993) Cephalic replacement for shoulder dystocia: present status and future role of the Zavanelli manoeuvre. Obstet Gynecol 82:847–855

Poggi SH, Spong CY, Allen RH (2003) Prioritizing posterior arm delivery during severe shoulder dystocia. Obstet Gynecol 101:1068–1072

Rouse DJ, Owen J (1999) Prophylactic caesarean delivery for fetal macrosomia diagnosed by means of ultrasonography – a Faustian bargain? Am J Obstet Gynecol 181:332–338

Royal College of Obstetricians and Gynaecologists (2012) Shoulder dystocia (green-top guideline no. 42). RCOG Press, London

Sandmire HF, DeMott RK (2003) Erb's palsy causation: a historical perspective. Birth 29:52–54

Sokol RJ, Blackwell SC (2003) American College of Obstetricians and Gynecologists. Shoulder dystocia (guideline no. 40). Int J Gynaecol Obstet 80:87–92

Verkuly DAA (2001) Symphysiotomies are an important option in the developed world. BMJ 323:809

World Health Organisation, Department of Reproductive Health and Research (2007) Shoulder dystocia (stuck shoulders). In: Managing complications in pregnancy and childbirth: guidelines for Midwives and for Doctors. WHO Press, Geneva, pp S83–S85

Wykes CB, Johnston TA, Paterson-Brown S, Johanson RB (2003) Symphysiotomy: a lifesaving procedure. BJOG 110:219–221

Retention of the After-Coming Head 4

4.1 Definition, Incidence and Main Risk Factors

Retention of the after-coming head refers to the rare situation in which there is difficulty in extracting the fetal head during vaginal breech delivery (Fig. 4.1). The incidence of breech presentation in labour varies according to gestational age, from about 23 % at 28 weeks to 3–4 % at term. The latter incidence depends also on local practices for the promotion of external cephalic version. The number of vaginal breech deliveries complicated by retention of the after-coming head is largely dependent on local policies of case selection for elective caesarean section. Footling or knee presentations, fetuses with estimated birth weights above 3800 g or below 1500 g and those with extended heads are common indications for caesarean section, but criteria may vary between centres. Some studies report retention of the after-coming head to occur in as much as 10 % of vaginal breeches, but the criteria used for the diagnosis are questionable.

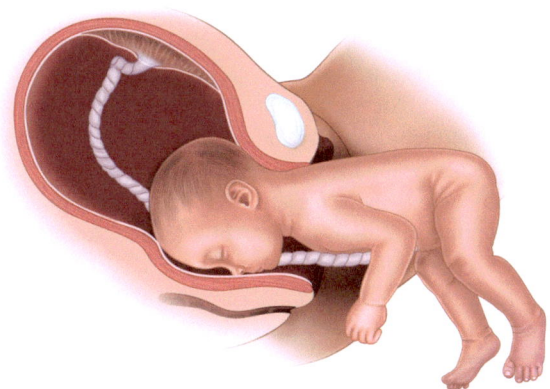

Fig. 4.1 Retention of the after-coming head

© Springer International Publishing Switzerland 2017
D. Ayres-de-Campos, *Obstetric Emergencies*,
DOI 10.1007/978-3-319-41656-4_4

Table 4.1 Risk factors for retention of the after-coming head

Fetal macrosomia or macrocephaly
Extended fetal neck
Reduced maternal pelvic diameters
Prolonged second stage of labour
Incompletely dilated cervix at the time of delivery
Rapid descent of the fetus in preterm delivery

Moulding of the fetal head to the birth canal is frequent during the course of labour in cephalic presentations, but there is little time for this to occur in breeches. In preterm fetuses head-to-pelvis ratios are higher, and this may allow the fetal pelvis to pass through an incompletely dilated cervix, while the head is later retained.

The risk factors for retention of the after-coming head are displayed in Table 4.1 and are mainly related to fetal head dimensions, flexion of the fetal neck and dimensions of the maternal pelvis. An extended fetal neck predisposes to retention because it increases the anteroposterior diameter of the head.

Currently, these risk factors are used mainly to select cases where elective caesarean section is proposed as the preferential mode of delivery, but in some centres this is proposed to all women with breech presentations at term or in labour.

Independently of these practices, healthcare professionals need to maintain competence in management of retention of the after-coming head, because they may always encounter it unexpectedly, particularly when women present in advanced labour with the breech already delivering.

4.2 Consequences

The main complication of fetal head retention is **acute hypoxia/acidosis**, due to umbilical cord compression between the fetal head and the surrounding maternal tissues, while the airway is still not in contact with air. Additional complications may arise from iatrogenic trauma caused by attempts to resolve the situation.

Perinatal mortality in some series reaches 4–8 % and is mainly due to hypoxia/acidosis and intracranial haemorrhage, but it is also related to the increased risk of malformations associated with breech presentation at term. **Perinatal morbidity** includes hypoxic-ischaemic encephalopathy; dislocation or fracture of cervical vertebrae; stretching/lacerations of the brachial-cephalic plexus and cervical muscles; dislocation of the lower jaw; fracture of the femur, humerus and clavicle; rupture of abdominal organs (spleen, liver, kidney, suprarenal glands); external genital lesions; meconium aspiration syndrome; infection; and neonatal sepsis.

Little is known about how long head retention may last before perinatal death or long-term injury occur. The situation providing the closest parallel for comparison is shoulder dystocia with coexisting nuchal cords (Chap. 3). Although there are no absolute certainties, less than 5 min of sustained cord compression is unlikely to put the fetus at risk, while a 5–9 min interval appears to be associated with mild short-term neurological dysfunction and full recovery, and more than 12 min causes substantial risk of permanent damage. These timings require adaptation when fetal oxygenation is previously compromised and when there is fetal growth restriction. Because of sustained cord occlusion, umbilical blood gas values may not reflect the severity of hypoxia/acidosis, and the occurrence of hypoxic-ischaemic encephalopathy will be the best predictor of long-term outcome.

Maternal morbidity arises mainly from the manoeuvres used for fetal extraction and includes vaginal lacerations, urethral and bladder injuries, vesical-vaginal and recto-vaginal fistulae, endometritis, postpartum sepsis, uterine rupture and postpartum haemorrhage.

4.3 Diagnosis

Retention of the after-coming head is established after there have been two or three unsuccessful attempts to extract the fetal head in a vaginal breech delivery. The most commonly used methods for this extraction are the Mauriceau-Smellie-Veit and the Bracht manoeuvres (see below).

4.4 Clinical Management

4.4.1 Guaranteeing the Conditions for a Safe Vaginal Breech Delivery

When important risk factors for retention of the after-coming head exist (Table 4.1), caesarean section should be proposed at all stages of labour before delivery of the shoulders. In the remaining situations, it is important to guarantee the conditions for a safe vaginal breech delivery. In high-resource countries, this usually means **continuous cardiotocographic monitoring** (internal or external), **emptying the bladder** before delivery and assembling the **necessary material** for resolving the possible complications of vaginal breech delivery. It is useful to have a **large swab** on hand, to hold the fetal body when it is too slippery and to also hold the extremities and umbilical cord when applying the Piper forceps (see below). A **vaginal retractor** and an **appropriate forceps** (Piper forceps or similar) should also be kept on hand, in case they are needed.

If time allows and the mother requests this, epidural analgesia should be put in place. Venous catheterisation is routinely used in many centres, to anticipate the situations in which uterine relaxation or emergency caesarean section is required. For delivery, the largest reported experience is with the mother in lithotomy position and the lower part of the bed removed. The hands and knees position is used as an alternative in some centres, but more data is required to establish its safety in generalised settings. Routine episiotomy was recommended in the past for all cases of vaginal breech delivery, but an increasing number of centres have moved away from this practice.

4.4.2 Anticipate the Situation

The prodromal signs suggestive of impending head retention are a prolonged second stage of labour, descent of the breech during contractions followed by an immediate return to the previous station and rapid descent of a preterm fetus with still incomplete cervical dilatation. When these are identified, steps should be taken to summon an experienced healthcare team, in case retention of the after-coming head occurs.

4.4.3 Attempts to Deliver the Fetal Head

Release of the fetal head in vaginal breech deliveries is classically accomplished by the Mauriceau-Smellie-Veit or Bracht manoeuvres, with no robust evidence of the advantages of either.

For the **Mauriceau-Smellie-Veit** manoeuvre, one hand and forearm support the ventral part of the fetal body, while the second and third fingers are placed on the upper lip to depress the malar eminences and thus flex the neck. The second and fourth fingers of the contralateral hand are placed on the dorsal aspect of the shoulders, one on each side of the neck, and the 3rd finger pushes the occiput bone forward to flex the fetal neck. After the fetal neck is flexed, moderate downward traction is applied on the shoulders until the occipital region is observed. With an assistant applying continuous suprapubic pressure, the fetal body is then slowly raised to rotate the neck gently around the pubic symphysis in the direction of the maternal abdomen (Fig. 4.2).

In the **Bracht manoeuvre**, the fetal breech and thighs are grasped with two hands, flexing the lower limbs, and the hands are slowly lifted upwards and around the pubic symphysis to deliver the fetal head (Fig. 4.3). No traction should be applied during this movement, but continuous suprapubic pressure by an assistant is required. Some authors propose the use of this manoeuvre after the umbilicus is delivered, to extract the fetal shoulders and head, while others propose it only for head extraction.

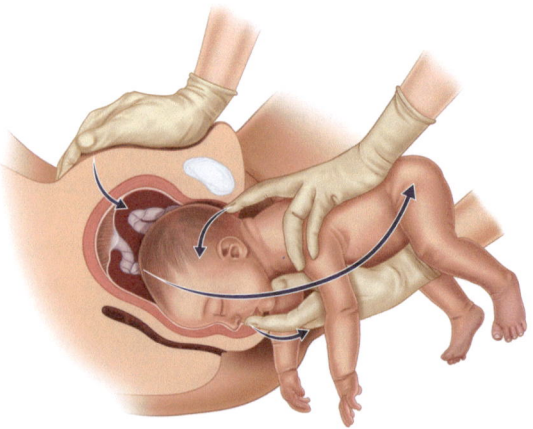

Fig. 4.2 The Mauriceau-Smellie-Veit manoeuvre

Fig. 4.3 The Bracht manoeuvre

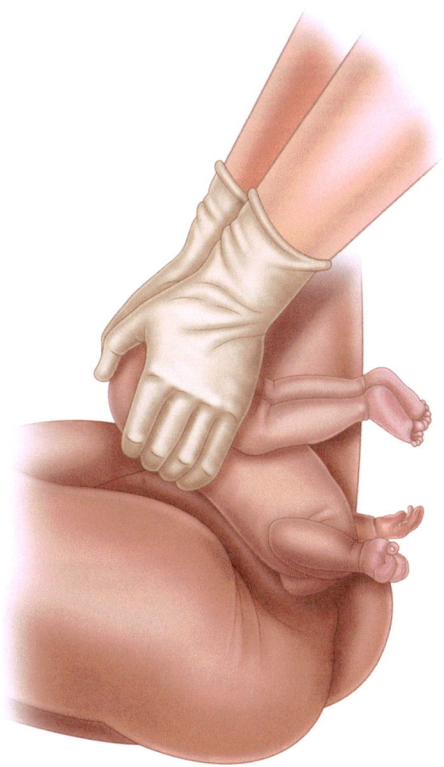

Both of these manoeuvres require particular care with mobilisation of fetal articulations and with pressure applied to the fetal thorax and abdomen, in order to avoid iatrogenic injury.

4.4.4 Clearly Verbalising the Diagnosis

It is important that all healthcare professionals present in the room are aware of the head retention, so that they can act accordingly. Therefore, the diagnosis needs to be clearly verbalised, without unnecessarily alarming the labouring woman and her companion.

4.4.5 Asking for Help

One of the first measures should be to summon **at least two midwives** and a **senior obstetrician**. In addition, a **neonatologist** and an **anaesthetist** should be called, the first one because neonatal resuscitation is likely to be needed and the second one because uterine relaxation may be required (see below).

4.4.6 McRobert's Position

Similarly to what occurs in shoulder dystocia (see Chap. 3), the McRobert's position straightens the lumbosacral angle and widens the anteroposterior diameter of the maternal pelvis, facilitating extraction of the fetal head. An additional attempt at head extraction with the Mauriceau-Smellie-Veit manoeuvre should be considered after adopting this position.

4.4.7 Episiotomy

If it is felt that the maternal perineum poses resistance to extraction of the fetal head, an episiotomy should be performed. This will also be useful for the application of forceps to the after-coming head.

4.4.8 Fetal Monitoring

When internal fetal heart rate monitoring is in place, the signal should continue to be acquired after the fetal body is released. With external fetal heart rate, the Doppler sensor located on the maternal abdomen will no longer pick up heart movements, but fetal monitoring can be continued by placing the Doppler sensor directly on the fetal thorax. Evaluating umbilical cord pulsatility may fail to provide a reliable measure of fetal heart rate, because of sustained cord compression.

4.4.9 Insertion of a Vaginal Retractor

Some guidelines recommend the temporary insertion of a vaginal retractor to push back the posterior vaginal wall and thus to allow oxygen to reach the fetal airways (Fig. 4.4). There is little evidence on the efficacy of this procedure, but it takes little time and is unlikely to cause harm.

4.4.10 Forceps to the After-Coming Head

The Piper forceps was specifically designed for managing retention of the after-coming head. However, when these forceps are unavailable, it is possible to use other types of forceps, such as Simpson's or Tarnier's.

To apply the Piper forceps, an assistant holds the fetal body, extremities and umbilical cord with two hands (or with a large swab) and raises these structures slightly to create space for inserting the forceps below (Fig. 4.5). The blades of the forceps are inserted one at a time, on each side of the head, guided by the contralateral hand. Once the blades are articulated, the fetal body is rested on the forceps, one of the executor's hands grabs the handle, and the contralateral hand is applied around the fetal shoulders, using a similar grip to that of the Mauriceau-Smellie-Veit

4.4 Clinical Management

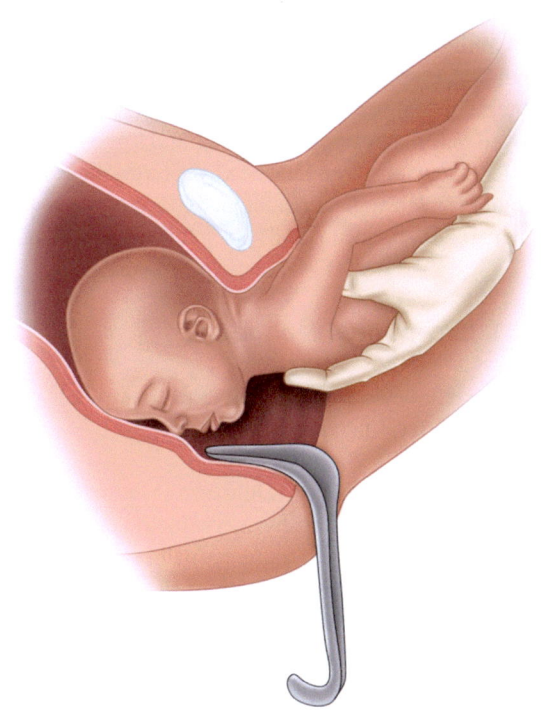

Fig. 4.4 Insertion of a vaginal retractor

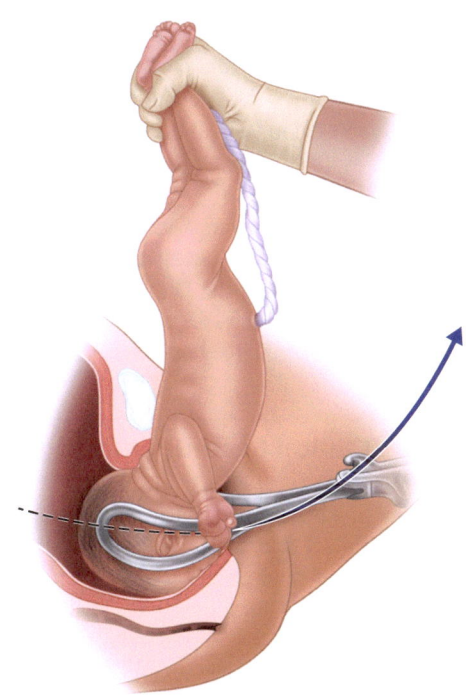

Fig. 4.5 Piper forceps applied and the trajectory of fetal head rotation

manoeuvre. Moderate traction is then applied to the forceps, initially slightly downwards until the fetal occiput is visible, and then to slowly rotate the fetal head around the pubic symphysis while at the same time an assistant applies continuous suprapubic pressure to flex and descend it. If a vaginal retractor is in place, this needs to be removed before applying traction on the forceps.

After extraction of the fetal head, the birth canal should be carefully inspected with a speculum or with vaginal retractors for lacerations of the cervix, vagina, urethra, rectovaginal septum, perineum and anal sphincter, which may require surgical correction.

4.4.11 Exceptional Manoeuvres

When the manoeuvres described above fail to deliver the after-coming head, exceptional manoeuvres need to be considered:

Lateral cervical incisions (Duhrssen incisions) – When retention of the fetal head is judged to be caused by incomplete cervical dilatation, as occurs in preterm deliveries, the cervical diameter can be increased by making two or three small incisions on the cervix. Sterilised rounded scissors are used to perform 1–2 cm cervical incisions at 2 and 10 o'clock and if necessary a third incision at 6 o'clock. These require surgical correction after the placenta is extracted.

Zavanelli's manoeuvre (replacement of the fetal shoulders in the maternal pelvis and vacuum-assisted caesarean delivery) – This manoeuvre should be performed in the operating theatre under general anaesthesia with halogenated agents. The shoulders are reintroduced one at a time into the vagina, and immediate caesarean section follows. A vacuum extractor is applied to the fetal head to release the remaining body while an assistant pushes the fetal pelvis up to help reinsert it into the vagina.

Symphysiotomy – This technique is described in detail in Chap. 3, and its use has been reported in a small number of cases of head retention. However, care must be taken, as it associated with important maternal morbidity in inexperienced hands.

Occasionally, it remains impossible to extract the fetal head in a timely fashion, despite all these efforts, and an adverse fetal outcome needs to be considered. Absence of heart sounds when the Doppler sensor is placed directly on the fetal thorax will confirm the diagnosis. The situation still requires resolution, but in these cases, the manoeuvres described above can be reattempted without the previous time pressure.

4.5 Clinical Records and Litigation Issues

The risk of adverse fetal outcome raises the possibility of litigation and the need for careful clinical records. It is important to document the time at which the fetal shoulders and fetal head were delivered, who were the healthcare professionals summoned, when they were called and when they arrived, and which manoeuvres were performed, when and by whom.

Umbilical blood gas values and Apgar scores should also be documented (see Chap. 2). Because of continued cord compression, pH values may not reflect the severity of fetal hypoxia/acidosis, so hypoxic-ischaemic encephalopathy will establish the best long-term prognosis in these cases. Strict adherence to guidelines, together with careful recording of events is required to avoid an adverse legal resolution.

MANAGEMENT OF RETENTION OF THE AFTER-COMING HEAD

Conditions for safe breech	Continuous CTG	☐
	Empty the bladder	☐
	Large swab, vaginal retractor, Piper forceps	☐
Anticipate the situation	Summon experienced team	
Diagnosis	Attempt Mauriceau-Smellie-Veit or Bracht maneuver	☐
	Verbalise the diagnosis	☐
Call for help	Two midwives	☐
	Senior obstetrician	☐
	Neonatologist	☐
	Anesthetist	☐
McRobert's position	Re-attempt Mauriceau-Smellie-Veit or Bracht	☐
Episiotomy (if needed)		☐
Fetal monitoring	Internal or external FHR on fetal thorax	☐
Place vaginal retractor		☐
Forceps application	Assistant lifts up fetus, extremities and cord	☐
	Apply blades, one at a time	☐
	Traction and suprapubic pressure	☐
	Inspection of the birth canal	☐
Exceptional maneuvers	Lateral cervical incisions	☐
	Zavanelli's maneuver	☐
	Symphysiotomy	☐
Clinical records	Cord blood gases and Apgar scores	☐
	Time of delivery of fetal shoulders and head	☐
	People called, at what time, and when they arrived	☐
	Maneuvers performed, when and by whom	☐

Suggested Reading

Collea JV (1981) The intrapartum management of breech presentation. Clin Perinatol 8:173

Gimovsky ML, Petrie RJ (1989) The intrapartum management of breech presentation. Clin Perinatol 16:975

Hannah ME, Hannah WJ, Hewson SA, Hodnett ED, Saigal S, Willan AR, for the Term Breech Trial Collaborative Group (2000) Planned caesarean section versus planned vaginal birth for breech presentation at term: a randomised multicentre trial. Lancet 356:1375–1383

Hickok DE, Gordon DC, Milberg JA et al (1992) The frequency of breech presentation by gestational age at birth: a large population-based study. Am J Obstet Gynecol 166:851

Mukhopadhyay S, Arulkumaran S (2002) Breech delivery. Best Pract Res Clin Obstet Gynaecol 16:31–42

Myers SA, Gleicher N (1987) Breech delivery: why the dilemma? Am J Obstet Gynaecol 156:6–10

Royal College of Obstetricians and Gynaecologists (2006) Practice guideline no. 20b. The management of breech presentation. RCOG Press, London

Society of Obstetricians and Gynecologists of Canada (2009) Practice guideline no 226. Vaginal delivery of breech presentation. J Obstet Gynaecol Can 31(6):557–566

Westrgren M, Grundsell H, Ingemarson I et al (1981) Hyperextension of the fetal head in breech presentation: a study with long-term follow-up. Br J Obstet Gynaecol 88:101

Part II

Predominantly Maternal Emergencies

Eclampsia 5

5.1 Definition, Incidence and Main Risk Factors

Hypertensive diseases of pregnancy remain a leading cause of maternal and perinatal mortality in both low- and high-resource countries, and eclampsia represents their most serious manifestation. Eclampsia is characterised by the occurrence of generalised tonic-clonic seizures (grand mal) in a woman who usually displays the typical symptoms, signs and laboratory findings of pre-eclampsia. The pathophysiologic mechanism behind eclamptic seizures remains incompletely understood, but endothelial lesion, exaggerated microvascular permeability, cerebral oedema and pericapillary haemorrhage are common findings.

The episode usually starts with a slight tremor of the facial muscles, shortly followed by a generalised tonic seizure of 15–20 s and then develops into generalised tonic-clonic seizures which may last over 1 min. The total duration of the episode rarely exceeds 90 s. Occasionally, seizures may recur rapidly with uninterrupted generalised contracture. No respiratory movements occur during tonic-clonic seizures, and this can have serious consequences on maternal and fetal oxygenation. When the episode terminates, there is a deep and noisy inspiration followed by a comatose state that is usually superficial and of variable duration, with slow recovery of consciousness. Subsequent agitation may develop, and the woman usually refers amnesia to the event. Transient cortical blindness and focal motor deficits may follow. Cerebral haemorrhage complicates 1–2 % of cases.

Eclampsia may occur during pregnancy (40–50 %), in labour (13–20 %) or in the postpartum period (28–40 %). With the implementation of policies for screening and early diagnosis of pre-eclampsia, as well as the prevention of seizures and prompt termination of pregnancy in cases of severe pre-eclampsia, the incidence of eclampsia has decreased dramatically over the last decades. In high-resource countries, pre-eclampsia is currently reported to occur in 2–8 % of pregnancies and eclampsia to complicate 0.2–0.3 % of these cases, for an overall incidence of 0.004–0.02 % of births. In many low- and medium-resource countries, the reported incidences of pre-eclampsia and eclampsia are much higher.

Table 5.1 Risk factors for pre-eclampsia and eclampsia	
	Primigravid
	Extremes of reproductive age
	Family history of pre-eclampsia
	Gestational or pre-existing diabetes
	Chronic hypertension or renal disease
	Multiple pregnancy
	Gestational trophoblastic disease
	Hereditary or acquired thrombophilia

The main risk factors for eclampsia are similar to those of pre-eclampsia and are listed in Table 5.1.

5.2 Complications

In high-resource countries, **maternal mortality** occurs in about 0.07 % of eclampsia cases, and the main causes are intracranial haemorrhage, acute pulmonary oedema and multi-organ failure. **Maternal morbidity** includes acute pulmonary oedema, disseminated intravascular coagulation, renal insufficiency and more rarely intracranial haemorrhage and rupture of subcapsular hepatic haematoma. Prolonged stay in intensive care units is frequently required in these cases.

Iatrogenic prematurity is frequent in severe pre-eclampsia and eclampsia and is responsible for the majority of **perinatal deaths**, which complicate about 26 % of eclampsia cases.

5.3 Diagnosis

Eclampsia is diagnosed when generalised tonic-clonic seizures are observed in a pregnant woman or a recent mother who usually displays the typical symptoms, signs and laboratory findings associated with pre-eclampsia.

The other major cause of generalised tonic-clonic seizures is epilepsy, and this can usually be identified by a history of previous episodes provided by a family member and/or a review of the patient's medication. When no other obvious cause exists, the episode should be treated as eclampsia, and other diagnoses can be later investigated, if there is inadequate response to treatment.

5.4 Clinical Management

5.4.1 Anticipate and Prevent the Situation

In patients with pre-eclampsia, the **prodromal symptoms** of severe frontal headache, continuous epigastric pain and visual complaints (blind spots, flashes, double vision and blurred vision) should alert to impending eclampsia. In patients with **severe pre-eclampsia** (papilloedema, hyperreflexia, platelets under $100 \times 10^9/l$,

5.4 Clinical Management

liver enzymes above 75 IU/l, oliguria, pulmonary oedema, nausea and vomiting), those with **severe hypertension in the context of pre-eclampsia** (blood pressure exceeding 160/110 mmHg) and those with prodromal symptoms, **intravenous magnesium sulphate** (see below) should be started to prevent seizures. Frequent re-evaluation of prodromal symptoms, blood pressure, laboratory results, together with seizure prevention with magnesium sulphate and termination of pregnancy if the situation deteriorates; these are the key elements for preventing eclampsia.

5.4.2 Ask for Help

The person(s) witnessing an eclamptic seizure should trigger a communication chain that results in the urgent summoning of **at least two midwives**, a **senior obstetrician**, and an **anaesthetist**. The anaesthetist will usually focus on maternal monitoring and maintenance of the airway, while the obstetrician will concentrate on starting magnesium sulphate and fetal monitoring. When the two specialities are not present, the person in charge needs to take all of these aspects into account.

5.4.3 Avoid Lesions During the Eclamptic Seizure

Restraining tonic-clonic movements is dangerous and confers no benefit to patients, so the recommended attitude during the seizure is to **remove all objects that may cause injury** and wait until it ends, which usually takes less than 90 s.

5.4.4 Left Lateral Safety Position, Inspect Airway and Monitor

When the seizure ends, the patient should be placed in **left lateral safety position** (Fig. 5.1) and the **airway quickly inspected for patency**. In a second step, oropharyngeal secretions may be aspirated if they are abundant, a Mayo tube inserted if the patient remains unconscious and breathing is made difficult by the tongue and **oxygen by mask** should be started at 8 l/min.

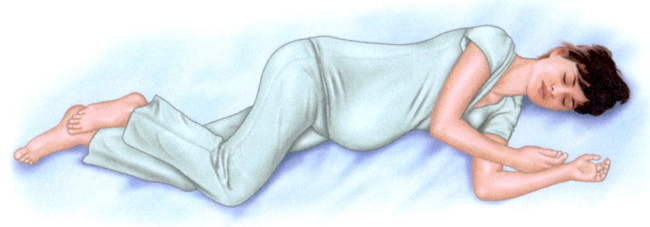

Fig. 5.1 Left lateral safety position

Maternal **heart rate** and **oxygen saturation** should be monitored continuously and blood pressure evaluated every 5 min. Maternal ventilation also requires frequent re-evaluation. If the woman is still pregnant, **continuous cardiotocography** should be put in place to evaluate fetal oxygenation. Eclamptic seizures usually condition a transitory fetal hypoxaemia and a short-lasting deceleration. However, severe pre-eclampsia may also be associated with chronic placental insufficiency and abruption, conditioning more serious fetal heart rate changes.

5.4.5 Prevention of New Seizures

During or shortly after an eclamptic seizure, it is important for one of the team members to gather all the necessary materials for vein catheterisation and magnesium sulphate infusion. In some centres, there are pre-prepared "**eclampsia boxes**" containing these materials, and they can be rapidly fetched. However, regular maintenance of these boxes needs to be assured.

After the seizure has stopped, **vein catheterisation** should be rapidly performed and the **loading dose of magnesium sulphate** started to avoid recurrences (Table 5.2).

5.4.6 Other Non-emergent Measures

After the acute response to eclampsia described above, the situation still requires continuous monitoring and further management. Blood should be drawn for **haemoglobin, platelet count, liver and renal function and coagulation studies. Bladder catheterisation** should be performed to measure **urine output**, important for fluid balance and for optimising magnesium sulphate treatment.

5.4.7 Decreasing Blood Pressure

When maternal blood pressure rises above **160/105 mmHg,** it becomes necessary to reduce it, because of increased risks of cerebral haemorrhage, cardiac insufficiency, myocardial infarction and placental abruption.

Table 5.2 Magnesium sulphate for the prevention of eclampsia and recurrent seizures

Loading dose	Maintenance dose
4 g magnesium sulphate IV over 5–20 min 2 vials of 10 ml magnesium sulphate at 20 % (2 g/10 ml) in 100 ml saline at 300–1200 ml/h	**1–3 g magnesium sulphate IV per hour** 8 vials of 10 ml magnesium sulphate at 50 % (5 g/10 ml) in 1000 ml saline at 25–75 ml/h

Labetalol is a quick-acting alpha- and beta-adrenergic antagonist, with little effect on brain and uterine perfusion. It can be given orally in a 200 mg tablet, which will usually result in a blood pressure fall within 30 min. The tablet can be repeated after 60 min, if needed. Fixed doses are then started, varying from 200 mg every 12 h to a maximum of 400 mg every 6 h. If there is no response to oral labetalol therapy or if the patient does not tolerate it, continuous intravenous infusion can be started by diluting one 100 mg/20 ml vial in 100 ml of saline (1 ml = 0.83 mg) and starting infusion at 50 ml/h, after which it is adjusted according to the blood pressure, to values between 24 and 192 ml/h. For hypertensive crises, an intravenous labetalol bolus of 20 mg can be given over the course of 1 min, implying the injection of 4 ml of a 100 mg/20 ml vial. The dose can be repeated every 10 min until a maximum dose of 200 mg is reached (10 boluses). This medication should be avoided in asthmatic women, and maternal heart rate should be maintained above 60 bpm.

Nifedipine is a relatively rapidly acting calcium channel blocker that can be administered orally in 10 or 20 mg tablets, given every 4–6 h. The sublingual route should be avoided, as it is associated with marked maternal hypotension and decreased placental perfusion. The classical contraindication to associate nifedipine with magnesium sulphate, because of the risk of hypotension and pulmonary oedema, has not been confirmed in several recent case series.

Hydralazine is a peripheral vasodilator that can be given intravenously in a 5 mg bolus over the course of 5 min. This implies injecting 0.25 ml of a 1 ml vial (20 mg/1 ml). The dose can be repeated every 20 min, for a maximum daily dose of 20 mg. Alternatively, a continuous intravenous infusion can be started at 0.5–10 mg/h. This is accomplished by diluting one 1 ml vial (20 mg/1 ml) in 100 ml of saline (1 ml = 0.2 mg) and infusing it at 2.5–50 ml/h, to a maximum daily dose of 20 mg. Tachycardia, headache, nausea and sweating are common side effects. Preloading or co-administration of 500 ml of intravenous crystalloid fluid reduces the risk of severe hypotension seen with intravenous hydralazine and should be considered if delivery has not yet occurred.

During antihypertensive treatment, blood pressure should initially be monitored every 5 min, and the interval is then spaced according to treatment results. The goal is to maintain systolic blood pressure between 140 and 150 mmHg and diastolic blood pressure between 80 and 100 mmHg. Lower diastolic blood pressures may put cerebral and uterine perfusion at risk.

5.4.8 Recurrent Seizures

When recurrent seizures occur after magnesium sulphate infusion is initiated, an intravenous bolus of 2–4 g of magnesium sulphate can be given over the course of 5 min. If seizures persist, the diagnosis of eclampsia should be reconsidered and a re-evaluation carried out with the help of a neurologist. Intravenous diazepam is less efficient than magnesium sulphate for preventing recurrent seizures and reducing maternal mortality, but is a possible alternative, given in a 5 mg bolus over the course of 5 min and repeated if necessary to a maximum of 20 mg. Prolonged use of diazepam should be avoided, as it is associated with an increased risk of maternal death and neonatal respiratory depression. If seizures persist, intubation and ventilation remain as a last resource, in an intensive care unit setting.

5.4.9 Maintenance Dose of Magnesium Sulphate

The maintenance dose of magnesium sulphate should be started as soon as the loading dose has finished, and the infusion is maintained at least until 24 h after birth or after the last seizure, whichever occurs latest (Table 5.2).

Magnesium sulphate is a drug with a low safety margin and is capable of conditioning serious side effects, such as muscular paralysis, central nervous system depression and cardiac arrest. It is predominantly excreted by the kidneys, so oliguria has a major impact on plasma concentrations. Treatment with magnesium sulphate requires frequent monitoring of urine output, respiratory frequency and the patellar reflex, evaluations that should be performed at least every 4 h. If urine output drops below 30 ml/h, patellar reflexes become week and/or respiratory frequency is under 16 cycles/min, serum magnesium levels should be evaluated, and the measures described in Table 5.3 should be undertaken. In many centres, serum magnesium levels are also routinely measured at 2, 6 and 12 h after the start of treatment.

About 25 % of women report side effects with intravenous magnesium sulphate, the most common of which is flushing.

Table 5.3 Serum magnesium, expected clinical findings, interpretation and management

Magnesium (mg/l)	Clinical findings	Interpretation and management
1.5–2.5	None	Subtherapeutic levels
4–8	None	Therapeutic levels
9–12	Loss of patellar reflex, sedation, nausea, diplopia, respiration <12 cycles/min, O_2 sat <95 %	Stop infusion, give oxygen and quantify serum magnesium. Re-evaluate every 15 min. If no improvement – calcium gluconate 1 g (1 g/10 ml) IV over 10 min. After recovery, restart infusion at half dose
15–17	Muscle paralysis, respiratory arrest, prolonged QRS	Calcium gluconate 1 g (1 g/10 ml) IV over 10 min, intubation, intensive care
30–35	Cardiac arrest	Cardiac massage, intubation and ventilation, calcium gluconate 1 g (1 g/10 ml) IV over 10 min, intensive care

5.4.10 Fluid Balance

The increased vascular permeability found in women with pre-eclampsia increases the risk of acute pulmonary oedema, cardiac insufficiency and cerebral oedema. For these reasons, total **fluid volume should not exceed 83 ml/h** (2 l in 24 h) except if there are other sources of fluid loss, such as haemorrhage. **Colloids should not be administered** except in life-saving situations. Oliguria does not usually require additional measures beyond fluid adjustments to the established limits, as it will revert spontaneously 36–48 h after delivery.

5.4.11 Thromboprophylaxis

Women with severe pre-eclampsia and eclampsia are at increased risk of venous thrombosis, so compression stockings and prophylactic doses of low molecular weight heparin need to be considered according to local protocols, until the patient is fully mobile.

5.4.12 Evaluation of Laboratory Results and Fetal Evaluation

The urgency of pregnancy termination and the method of delivery depend on the clinical stability of the situation; on laboratory results depicting the severity of pre-eclampsia, particularly the degree of thrombocytopenia and liver enzymes; and on the fetal condition. Pre-eclampsia may be associated with chronic placental insufficiency, so fetal ultrasound is required to evaluate fetal growth, amniotic fluid volume and umbilical and cerebral blood flow.

5.4.13 Programming Birth

Pregnancy termination and placental extraction constitute the only known cure for pre-eclampsia. Recurrence of seizures after the initial eclampsia event poses unacceptable health risks to the mother, so delivery needs to be programmed as soon as blood pressure is stabilised and laboratory results are evaluated, independently of gestational age or of fetal prognosis. If prodromal signs have disappeared, blood pressure has been controlled, only mild changes are present in laboratory results and conditions to **induce labour** are favourable, this should be attempted with the aim of achieving **delivery within 8–12 h**. Both oxytocin and prostaglandins may be used in conjunction with magnesium sulphate, but care must be taken not to exceed the recommended hourly fluid replacement volume. Continuous maternal monitoring and cardiotocography should be maintained throughout the full course of labour.

Epidural analgesia may be used for pain relief if the platelet count is above $80 \times 10^9/l$. A slight decrease in blood pressure should be expected in these situations, but fluid preload is not recommended. Before 32 weeks, the Bishop score is seldom favourable, and the success rate of induction is low. When cervical characteristics are adverse and delivery is not expected to occur within 8–12 h or if there are other obstetric contraindications to vaginal delivery, the benefits of **elective caesarean section** should be explained to the patient and family. Both regional and general anaesthesia may be used for surgery, and the patient's platelet count needs to be taken into consideration.

When eclampsia occurs between 24 and 34 weeks of gestation, a **course of corticosteroids** should be administered as soon as possible. The neonatologist should be contacted in anticipation of an iatrogenic preterm delivery. Waiting for the full course of corticosteroids is usually not recommended, but there are reported benefits from partial courses. Magnesium sulphate may cause hypotension, hypotonia, respiratory depression and reduced suction reflex in newborns, so the neonatologist needs to be informed of this medication.

After delivery, it is prudent to transfer the woman to an intensive care unit until the haemodynamic, neurological and laboratory situation are stabilised.

5.5 Clinical Records and Litigation Issues

Eclampsia may be associated with adverse maternal and perinatal outcomes, so it is important to document the names of the healthcare professionals who were called, when this occurred and when they arrived, as well as who was involved in the decisions, when they were taken and who performed which procedures.

A frank explanation of the situation to the patient and to her family is important to avoid much of the suspicion, disinformation and misunderstanding that lead to litigation. When the latter occurs, strict adherence to existing guidelines and careful recording of events are important to guarantee a favourable legal outcome.

MANAGEMENT OF ECLAMPSIA

Anticipate and prevent	Severe PE or prodromes - start magnesium sulphate	☐
During seizure	Ask for help: 2 midwives, obstetrician, anaesthetist	☐
	Remove dangerous objects nearby	☐
	Get eclampsia box	☐
	Wait for seizure to pass	☐
After seizure	Left lateral safety position	☐
	Quickly evaluate airway patency	☐
	If necessary aspirate secretions, Mayo tube, O_2	☐
Monitoring	Continuous HR, O_2 sat; frequent BP and Resp Freq	☐
	Continuous CTG	☐
Prevention of recurrences	Catheterise peripheral vein	☐
	Start loading dose of magnesium sulphate	☐
Non-emergent measures	Draw blood for Hg, Plt, Coag, liver+renal function	☐
	Catheterise bladder and measure urine output	☐
	Antihypertensive medication if necessary	☐
	Start maintenance dose of magnesium sulphate	☐
	Limit fluid replacement	☐
	Thromboprophylaxis	☐
	Corticoids and contact neonatology if necessary	☐
	Evaluate lab tests, ultrasound	☐
Decide delivery	Vaginal examination	☐
	Labour induction or c-section	☐
Clinical records	People called, at what time, and when they arrived	☐
	Decisions taken, when and by whom	☐
	Procedures performed, when and by whom	☐

Suggested Reading

Duley L, Gülmezoglu AM, Henderson-Smart DJ, Chou D (2010) Magnesium sulphate and other anticonvulsants for women with pre-eclampsia. Cochrane Database Syst Rev (11):CD000025

Duley L, Meher S, Jones L (2013) Drugs for treatment of very high blood pressure during pregnancy. Cochrane Database Syst Rev (3):CD001449

National Institute for Health and Clinical Excellence (2011) Hypertension in pregnancy – the management of hypertensive disorders during pregnancy. RCOG Press, London

Tuffnell D (2003) Pre-eclampsia and eclampsia. In: Johanson R, Cox C, Grady K, Howell C (eds) Managing obstetric emergencies and trauma: the MOET course manual. RCOG Press, London, pp 151–70

Postpartum Haemorrhage

6.1 Definition, Incidence and Main Risk Factors

Postpartum haemorrhage occurs more frequently in the first 2 h after delivery and is classified as **early or primary postpartum haemorrhage** (i.e. occurring in the first 24 h after birth). Late or secondary postpartum haemorrhage (appearing after the first 24 h) is outside the aim of this chapter.

There is no worldwide agreement on the definitions of postpartum haemorrhage and major postpartum haemorrhage. Some define **postpartum haemorrhage** as blood loss exceeding 500 ml and **major postpartum haemorrhage** as blood loss exceeding 1000 ml. Others define postpartum haemorrhage as blood loss exceeding 500 ml in vaginal deliveries and exceeding 1000 ml at caesarean section. The limitation of all these definitions is the difficulty in quantifying blood loss accurately, particularly in vaginal deliveries. Collector bags can be used for this purpose, but blood frequently falls outside; amniotic fluid and urine may be collected and both will affect quantification. Weighing of swabs is routinely performed in some centres, but the practice is time-consuming and not widely disseminated, and similar inaccuracies to those referred for collector bags may occur. The most widely used alternative is visual estimation of blood loss, but this has well-known limitations, although improved accuracy may be achieved with visual aids, where the appearance of different blood quantity losses is depicted on photographs/drawings (Fig. 6.1). An additional problem arises from the fact that small women and those with pre-existing anaemia may decompensate with lesser quantities of blood loss.

Another definition of postpartum haemorrhage is a reduction in the haematocrit exceeding 10 %, but routine blood analysis before and after birth is rarely practised in low-risk labours, where the majority of complications occur. The need for blood transfusion is an alternative criterion, but it is used mainly in research settings, it leaves out less severe cases of haemorrhage, and transfusion criteria may vary between centres.

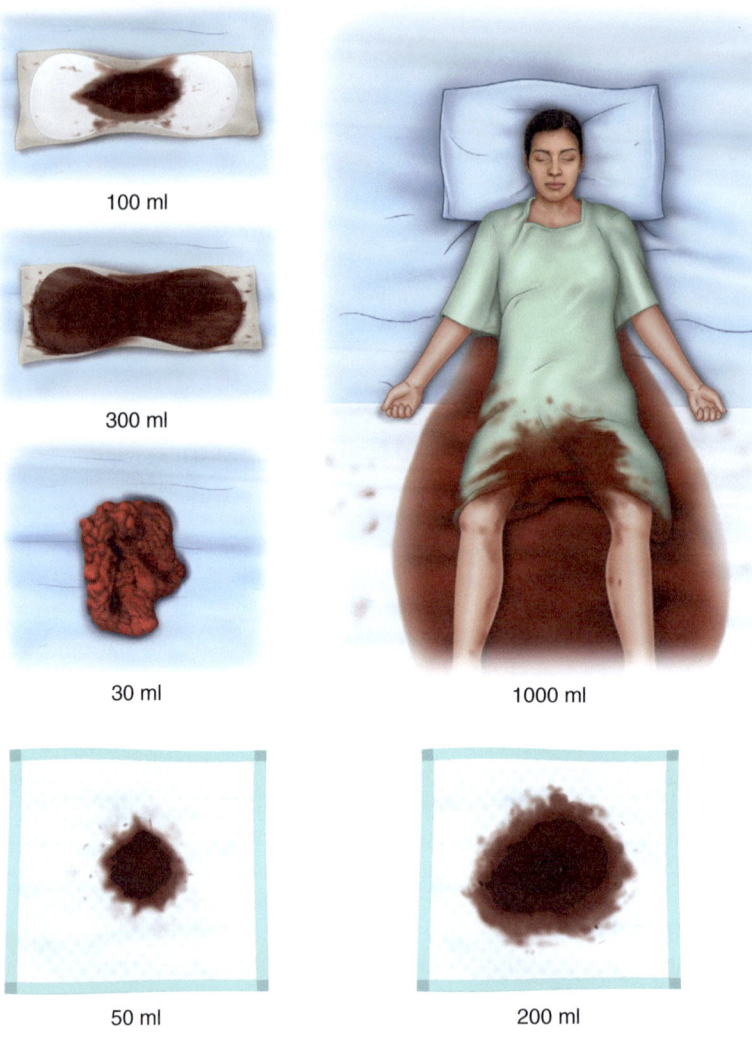

Fig. 6.1 Quantification of blood loss based on drawings

6.1 Definition, Incidence and Main Risk Factors

From a clinical point of view, the most important factor to define **postpartum haemorrhage** is the one that should trigger a response from the healthcare team. In the majority of situations, this occurs because **profuse and/or persistent genital bleeding** is witnessed to occur spontaneously after birth or when uterine massage is performed. Bleeding may be mild and rapidly reversible, so it is important to separate the concept of **major postpartum haemorrhage**, where more complex interventions need to be considered. **Blood loss exceeding 1000 ml or a heart rate approaching the systolic blood pressure** is probably the most useful criteria, from a clinical point of view. The "shock index", defined as the heart rate divided by systolic blood pressure, is used in other areas of Medicine and has recently been applied to postpartum haemorrhage. It is considered abnormal when exceeding 0.9.

The three major causes of early postpartum haemorrhage are **uterine atony**, which is responsible for about 70–80 % of cases, **genital tract lesions** accounting for 10–15 % of cases and **retained placental tissue**. Partial placental retention is usually associated with recurring uterine atony and haemorrhage. **Abnormally adherent placenta** (accreta, increta and percreta) is normally associated with haemorrhage when attempts are made to remove the placenta, and its incidence has been increasing in some parts of the world because of escalating caesarean section rates. Rarer causes of postpartum haemorrhage are **uterine inversion, uterine rupture** and **maternal bleeding disorders**. Uterine inversion is thought to be caused mainly by mismanagement of the third stage of labour, namely by excessive pressure on the uterine fundus, premature traction on the umbilical cord or excess traction during manual removal of an abnormally adherent placenta. Less frequently it occurs after an episode of coughing or vomiting during the third stage of labour.

The incidence of early postpartum haemorrhage varies widely, depending on the criteria used for the diagnosis, the population studied and the methods used for prevention, but it is reported to occur in 2–10 % of all deliveries. The most important risk factors are listed in Table 6.1, but many cases occur in women where these are not present.

Table 6.1 Risk factors for postpartum haemorrhage	
	High parity
	High uterine volume – multiple pregnancy, macrosomia, polyhydramnios
	Caesarean delivery and instrumental vaginal delivery
	Prolonged or precipitate labour
	Labour induction and acceleration
	Placental abruption
	Uterine leiomyomas and malformations
	Maternal bleeding disorders
	Corioamnionitis
	Placenta praevia and abnormally adherent placenta
	Pre-eclampsia
	Amniotic fluid embolism
	Previous postpartum haemorrhage

6.2 Consequences

Postpartum haemorrhage remains an important cause of **maternal mortality**, in both low- and high-resource countries. In European countries, maternal deaths due to postpartum haemorrhage occur in about 0.003 % of all births, and this incidence has not changed significantly over the last 30 years.

Less is known about **maternal morbidity** associated with postpartum haemorrhage, but most of it is related to the side effects of treatment. Some surgical procedures are associated with loss of fertility (conservative treatments and hysterectomy), infectious morbidity, urologic lesion and intensive care unit stay. Other complications are associated with allergic reactions to medication, colloids and blood replacement products. Birth canal lacerations may also occur as a consequence of mechanical treatments, but these seldom have long-term consequences. Decreased perfusion of the pituitary gland for prolonged periods of time has been associated with secondary panhypopituitarism (Sheehan's syndrome), but this complication is currently very rare in high-resource countries.

6.3 Diagnosis

Postpartum haemorrhage can be defined as **profuse and/or persistent genital bleeding** occurring spontaneously after birth or when uterine massage is performed. The diagnosis may be triggered by routine clinical re-evaluation, maternal complaints of dizziness and loss of vision, maternal paleness or by the detection of tachycardia or hypotension. The main clinical usefulness of this definition is that it constitutes a trigger for action from the healthcare team.

The diagnosis of **major postpartum haemorrhage** implies the same findings, but in addition **blood loss exceeds 1000 ml** (by quantification or visual estimation) or **maternal heart rate approaches systolic blood pressure** (the shock index exceeds 0.9).

6.4 Clinical Management

Management of postpartum haemorrhage involves two major components – support of maternal circulation/oxygenation and treatment of the underlying cause. When an anaesthetist and an obstetrician are present in the room, the responsibility for these two aspects is usually divided among them. In the remaining situations, the person in charge needs to take care of both.

6.4.1 Anticipating the Situation

When the risk factors listed in Table 6.1 are identified, increased surveillance usually allows earlier diagnosis and intervention. Continuous monitoring of maternal pulse and blood pressure should be considered in the first stages of any abnormal genital bleeding, in addition to frequent re-evaluation of haemorrhage and uterine contracture.

6.4.2 Clearly Verbalising the Diagnosis

It is important that the whole team of healthcare professionals is aware of the diagnosis of postpartum haemorrhage, so that they can act accordingly, and therefore this needs to be clearly verbalised, without unnecessarily alarming the labouring woman and her companion.

6.4.3 Asking for Help

One of the first measures should be to summon urgently **at least two midwives**, a **senior obstetrician** and an **anaesthetist**. As stated above, the presence of an anaesthetist guarantees a safer management of basic circulatory and respiratory functions, as well as fluid balance. Care is however needed to maintain good communication between both sides at all times, so that there is coordinated management of the situation.

6.4.4 Initial Evaluation of the Cause of Haemorrhage

A quick evaluation needs to be carried out to establish the most likely cause of haemorrhage. This involves assessment of uterine contracture to diagnose uterine atony, a speculum evaluation to detect lacerations of the birth canal and a re-evaluation of the placenta to establish whether it is complete (no missing cotyledons on the maternal side, no lacerated vessels on the placental margin on the fetal side). Abnormally adherent placenta is usually diagnosed when placental extraction fails, and uterine inversion is diagnosed by bimanual examination. The rarer causes of uterine rupture and maternal bleeding disorders are usually considered only after the initial measures for treatment of postpartum haemorrhage have failed.

6.4.5 Support of Maternal Circulation and Oxygenation

6.4.5.1 Venous Catheterisation and Blood Volume Replacement
One of the first measures should be to guarantee adequate access for fluid perfusion, by **catheterising a vein with a large bore catheter** (14G or 16G). If major postpartum haemorrhage is identified, a second vein should be catheterised and at the same time blood collected for full blood count, coagulation studies and cross-matching. **Fluid replacement with crystalloids** (saline, Ringer's lactate) at high perfusion speeds should follow, avoiding dextrose solutions as they may worsen acidosis.

About three litres of crystalloids are required to replace one litre of blood loss, because of loss to the extravascular space. In previously healthy women, a 1.5 l blood loss can usually be compensated just with the use of crystalloids. With further loss, replacement with colloids and blood products needs to be considered (see below).

6.4.5.2 Maternal Monitoring
Continuous monitoring of maternal **heart rate** and **oxygen saturation** should be started promptly and **blood pressure** measured every 5–10 min. Consideration should also be given to **electrocardiographic monitoring**, particularly with major postpartum haemorrhage or when there is loss of consciousness.

6.4.5.3 Bladder Catheterisation and Measurement of Urinary Output
Bladder catheterisation is needed to measure urinary output, which should be kept above 30 ml/h, and to allow more effective external uterine massage (see below).

6.4.5.4 Maintain Maternal Oxygen Supply to the Brain
It is important to guarantee adequate oxygen supply to the brain, and for this the woman should be placed in a slight **head-down position** or alternatively her legs raised to increase venous return. **Oxygen** should be administered by face mask, starting at 30%, 10–15 l/min, and thereafter adapting according to oxygen saturation levels.

6.4.5.5 Decision to Start Colloids
When blood loss exceeds 1.5 l or there is difficulty in maintaining normal maternal blood pressure with crystalloids, administration of colloids needs to be considered. The latter includes albumin, dextran, gelatin and hydroxyethylamide. These substances assure a higher intravascular volume and some improve oxygen transport in the microcirculation, but they all carry a small risk of anaphylaxis. The frequency of severe reactions (shock, cardiorespiratory arrest) is 0.003 % for albumin, 0.008 % for dextran, 0.038 % for gelatin and 0.006 % for hydroxyethylamide. Colloid volumes exceeding 1000–1500 ml per day may also affect coagulation tests.

6.4.5.6 Decision to Administer Blood Products
Administration of blood products should be considered when haemorrhage persists and is approaching 2000 ml. It is usually also considered when there is prolonged haemodynamic instability or a low haemoglobin count. The main objective is to recover oxygen transport capacity, but there are also haemodynamic and clotting benefits. In a shared decision with the hospital blood bank, 2–4 units of packed red blood cells may be transfused initially. All obstetric units must have access to blood from universal donors (O negative blood) in less than 30 min, but usually there is time for cross-matching and individualised transfusion. There is currently no consensus on the ideal balance between transfusion of packed red cells and fresh frozen plasma, but it is prudent to administer at least one unit of fresh frozen plasma for each 4 units of packed red cells, in order to prevent consumption coagulopathy.

Additional blood transfusions, including cryoprecipitate, platelets and recombinant factor VIIa, are usually decided in coordination with the hospital blood bank, and serial evaluations of haemoglobin and coagulation tests are required to guide decisions.

6.4.5.7 Maintain Body Temperature
In hypovolemic shock, low body temperature will contribute to peripheral hypoperfusion and tissue damage. This can be reduced by maintaining normal body temperature and by administering previously warmed fluids.

6.4.6 Treatment of Uterine Atony

6.4.6.1 Initial Measures
The finding of a non-contracted uterus after placental delivery should lead to immediate **external uterine massage** in order to stimulate contraction. Previous **catheterisation of the bladder** facilitates this procedure and also allows measurement of urine output (see above).

6.4.6.2 Medical Treatment
The options available for medical treatment of uterine atony are displayed in Table 6.2. Regardless of whether or not it has been previously used for the prevention of postpartum haemorrhage, **oxytocin** should be the first-line treatment for uterine atony. It is preferably administered intravenously in rapid infusion, but can also be given by slow 10 IU intravenous bolus, although the latter has been associated with rare cases of severe maternal hypotension. If the intravenous route is not available, successful treatment of uterine atony with intramyometrial administration of 10 IU oxytocin has been reported in a small number of cases, by transcervical injection at 2 and 10 o'clock.

Uterine massage, bladder catheterisation and intravenous oxytocin resolve the majority of cases of uterine atony. There is little scientific evidence on which to base the order of subsequent treatments, so it depends mostly on local experience. **Rectal misoprostol** appears to be effective and safe, having as contraindications inflammatory bowel disease and a history of previous allergy to the drug. Transient hyperthermia may occur, but no measures are usually required to treat it. **Other**

Table 6.2 Uterotonic agents used for the medical treatment of uterine atony

Oxytocin 20 IU in 500 ml of saline, in IV perfusion at 250 ml/h
Prostaglandins:
Misoprostol 800–1000 μg rectal
Sulprostone 1 mg in 500 ml of saline, in IV perfusion at 125 ml/h, which can be increased up to 500 ml/h. After contracture, it is reduced to the initial dose
Carboprost (15-methyl prostaglandin F2 alpha) 0.25 mg IM, repeated every 15 min for a maximum of 8 doses

prostaglandins are available in some countries and have asthma, cardiac disease, hypertension and diabetes as contraindications.

6.4.6.3 Mechanical Treatments

Bimanual uterine compression is a simple procedure that generally controls bleeding from uterine atony and other intrauterine causes (Fig. 6.2). A hand is placed on the abdomen over the uterine fundus, and the contralateral one is inserted in the vagina to compress the cervix and uterus against the abdominal hand. Pressure should be sustained to collapse bleeding vessels and to promote coagulation in the placental bed. The procedure may not be applicable in some women, if it causes unreasonable pain or discomfort. The main difficulty resides in the executor's capacity to maintain sustained pressure for long periods of time, so frequent substitution may be required. It may also be used as a temporary measure to control bleeding, while other treatments are being considered or prepared.

Uterine balloon tamponade has gained popularity in the last decades and can be performed with devices especially developed for postpartum haemorrhage, the Bakri (Fig. 6.3) and Ebb balloons, or those adapted from other settings, the gastric part of the Sengstaken-Blakemore balloon (developed for oesophageal haemorrhage), the Rusch balloon (developed for bladder haemorrhage) or a condom adapted to a Foley catheter. The balloon is introduced through the cervix with a guiding hand, or using a speculum and sponge forceps, and filled with saline (ideally warmed up to 37 °C) until it is felt or seen to slightly dilate the cervix. The amount of fluid varies according to uterine dimensions, but is usually around 300–500 ml. Prophylactic antibiotics should be started and the balloon removed 12–24 h later. The reported success rate with this technique is around 85–90 %.

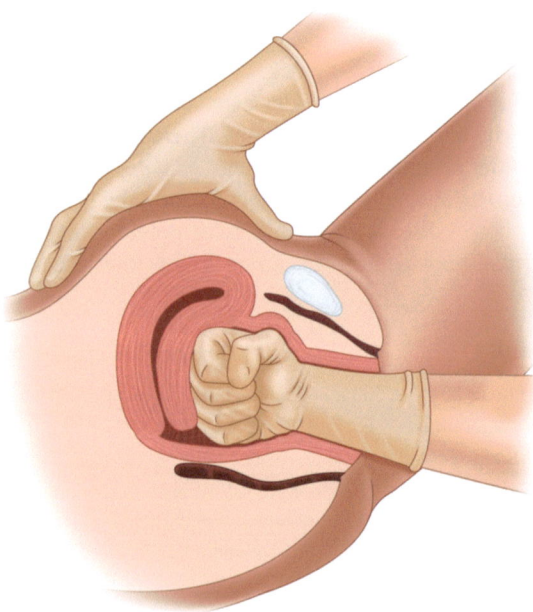

Fig. 6.2 Bimanual uterine compression

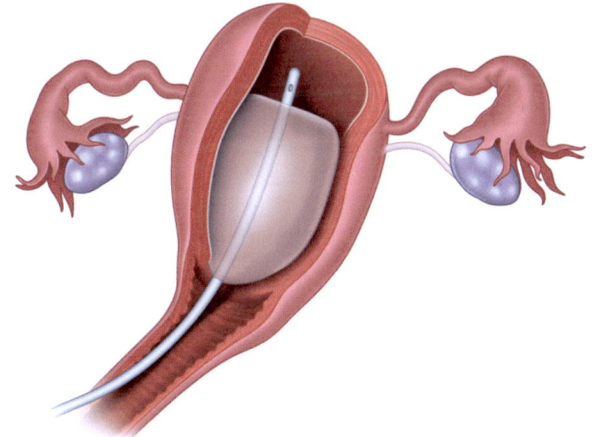

Fig. 6.3 Uterine tamponade with the Bakri balloon

In centres where there is an experienced intervention radiologist, **uterine artery embolisation** is another option. Angiography may be used to identify the bleeding vessels and to define the best strategy for embolisation. A catheter is then introduced into the femoral artery under local anaesthesia and inserted under fluoroscopic control until the tip lies at the root of the contralateral uterine artery. Embolisation may be performed with gelatin sponge pledgets, microspheres of polyvinyl alcohol or tri-acryl gelatin microspheres, all of which are absorbed in about 10 days. The complication rate depends on local experience, but is reported in about 5 % of cases. It includes fever, deep vein thrombosis, pancreatitis, infection, uterine necrosis, vascular perforation and femoral artery occlusion. Several observational studies report success rates of 90–95 % and cases of viable subsequent pregnancies.

In low-resource settings, **antishock garments** and **aortic pressure** may be used as temporary measures to reduce bleeding and the resulting haemodynamic instability, allowing patient transfer or the consideration of other treatments. Aortic pressure is performed by placing a hand in the midline above the uterus and exerting continuous downward pressure with the heel of the hand. These measures are seldom required in high-resource countries.

6.4.6.4 Surgical Treatments

When bleeding does not stop with the medical and/or mechanical methods described above, consideration must be given to moving the patient to the operating theatre and preparing for laparotomy.

Several **compression sutures** have been described, and they are most successful when intraoperative manual uterine compression results in cessation of bleeding. The **B-Lynch** suture (Fig. 6.4, left) is perhaps the most widely used, with a reported success rate of around 90 %. A pair of absorbable sutures is symmetrically placed on either side of the midline, but a second pair may be needed in large uteri. The B-Lynch suture was originally described for cases where there was a caesarean incision, and a modification described by **Hayman** may be used when the uterus is

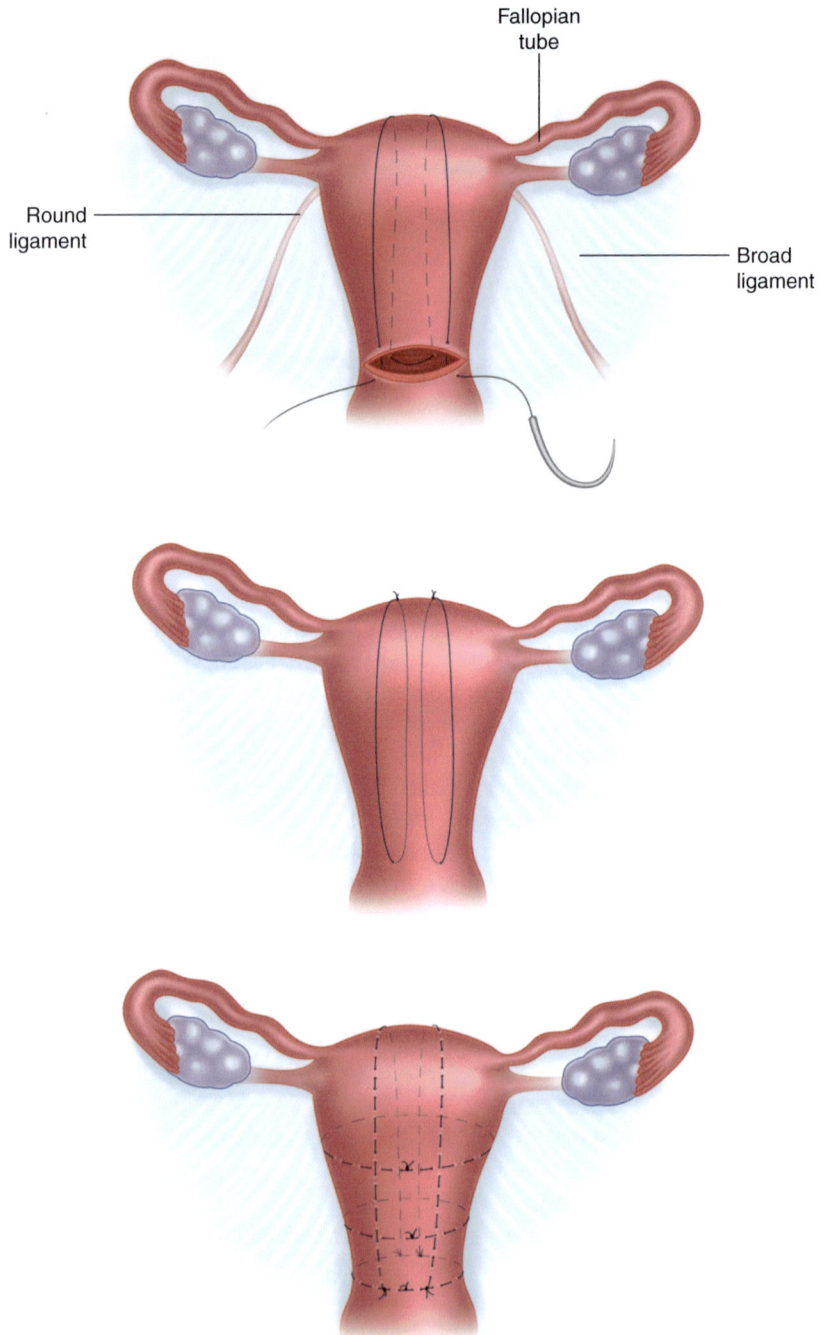

Fig. 6.4 The B-Lynch (*top*), the Hayman (*middle*) and the Pereira sutures (*bottom*)

intact (Fig. 6.4, centre). In addition to B-Lynch and Hayman sutures, transverse uterine **Pereira** sutures may be employed for increased compression, if necessary (Fig. 6.4, right).

For situations of continuous uterine bleeding from the lower uterine segment due to placenta praevia, **transfixing vertical sutures** are frequently successful in haemorrhage control (Fig. 6.5).

An alternative approach is **progressive uterine devascularisation**, involving a stepwise ligation of the ascending branch of one of the uterine arteries, followed by the contralateral one, the uterine branch of one of the ovarian arteries and the contralateral branch (Fig. 6.6). The sequence stops as soon as haemorrhage is controlled. For uterine artery ligation, the bladder is reflected downwards, a small opening is created in the broad ligament 2 cm below the level of a caesarean incision, and the needle is passed to transfix the myometrium about 2 cm from the lateral margin. Success rates are reported to be around 85%, and the technique is easier to execute than internal iliac (hypogastric) artery ligation. Uterine blood flow is maintained through anastomoses from the vesical and rectal arteries, and there is subsequent recanalisation of the uterine arteries. Cases of subsequent pregnancy have been reported.

Internal iliac (hypogastric) artery ligation has lost popularity over the last decades, as it requires the presence of a surgeon with experience in retroperitoneal dissection. Because of major collateral anastomoses present in the pelvis, the reported success rate is only 40-70%, and it is also associated with important maternal morbidity.

Peripartum hysterectomy is one of the last resorts in treatment of postpartum haemorrhage, and it should be considered when the patient does not desire future pregnancies and consents to the proposal or as a life-saving procedure when this situation is protected by law. Surgical technique is similar to that of hysterectomy performed for gynaecological reasons, but the pedicles are usually more thick, oedematous and vascular, so double clamping and ligation are usually preferable. Identifying the cervix may be difficult in these situations, and it is useful to insert a

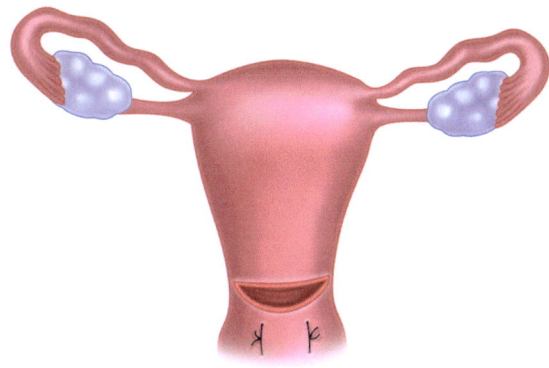

Fig. 6.5 Transfixing vertical sutures, used for bleeding from the lower uterine segment

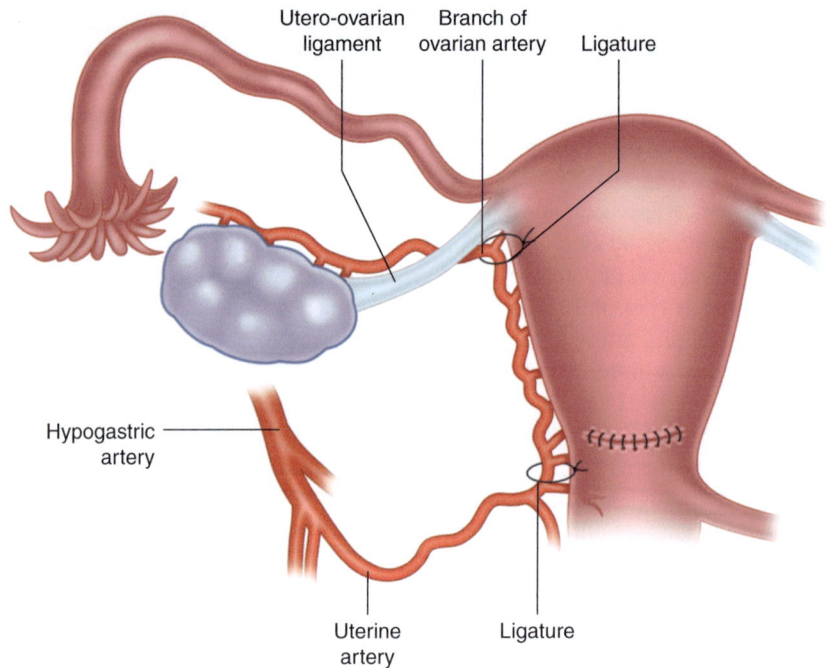

Fig. 6.6 Progressive uterine devascularisation

finger through the cervix into the vagina and hook it up to isolate the cervical rim. This will also guide the vaginal incision for total hysterectomy. Subtotal hysterectomy is usually easier to perform and is associated with less ureteral lesions. Recent studies report low mortality with the procedure, but morbidity and prolonged intensive care unit stay are frequent.

6.4.6.5 Pelvic Tamponade

When pelvic vessels continue to bleed after hysterectomy, pelvic tamponade with gauze inserted into a sterilised plastic bag and connected to a weight via the vaginal opening has been reported in a small number of cases (Fig. 6.7). Prophylactic antibiotics are started, and the bag is opened 24 h later to extract the gauze pads one by one, after which the bag is removed.

6.4.7 Treatment of Birth Canal Injuries

Birth canal injuries may be detected on the initial speculum examination or may need to be carefully searched in a later re-evaluation, motivated by persistent haemorrhage with the uterus firmly contracted. Adequate light, positioning and analgesia are required for this, together with vaginal retractors and a systematic approach to evaluate the cervix and vagina. Two ring forceps are usually used to explore the cervix, moving them alternatively to visualise the whole

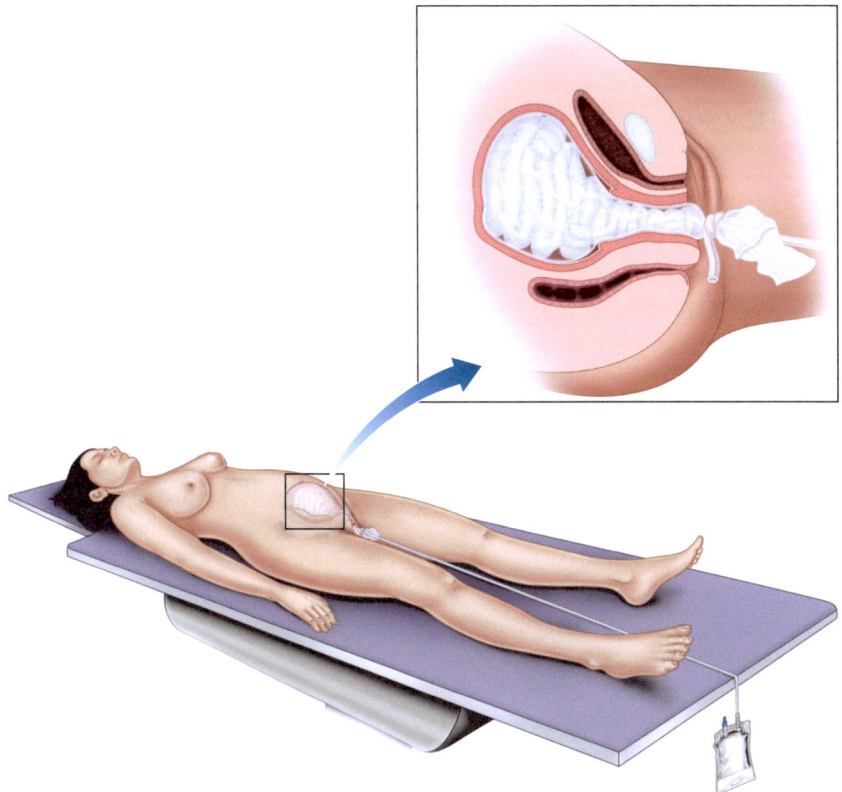

Fig. 6.7 Pelvic tamponade

circumference. Only **cervical lacerations** measuring more than 2–3 cm and those that are actively bleeding need to be repaired, using continuous absorbable suture and starting at the apex.

Vaginal wall lacerations should be visualised in their entire extension and corrected with a continuous absorbable suture. Any gushing arterial haemorrhage should be clamped and ligated individually. Subsequent vaginal packing with large swabs may be necessary to control minor bleeding, and when this occurs it is preferable to catheterise the bladder to avoid urinary retention. When located high in the vagina, lacerations may extend to the uterus and be associated with haematomas of the broad ligament and/or retroperitoneal space (see below).

Birth canal haematomas may be located in the vulva, vagina, broad ligament, ischial-rectal or retroperitoneal spaces and may form over the course of minutes or hours. They may occur in isolation or associated with vaginal lacerations and are caused by a vessel bleeding into a newly formed space. Small and non-expanding haematomas should be managed conservatively, with frequent re-evaluations of size and accompanying symptoms. Large or expanding haematomas require surgical drainage under anaesthesia. After removal of the blood and clots, bleeding vessels should be searched and ligated individually. If there is continued oozing, the space should be closed. Broad ligament and retroperitoneal haematomas can be diagnosed by ultrasound, computer tomography or magnetic resonance imaging. They are preferably treated conservatively, unless there is haemodynamic instability, infection or rapid expansion. Selective arterial embolisation by an intervention radiologist is currently the preferential method of treatment. Surgical treatment of retroperitoneal haematomas requires a surgeon with experience in the exploration of this space.

6.4.8 Treatment of Placental Retention

6.4.8.1 Complete Placental Retention
Complete retention of the placenta associated with haemorrhage requires prompt manual removal of the placenta under regional or general anaesthesia and subsequent uterine curettage if any fragments remain attached. This is followed by external uterine massage, prophylactic antibiotics and intravenous perfusion of uterotonic agents (Table 6.2) for at least 2 h. If a cleavage plane between the uterine wall and the placenta is not identified, this establishes the diagnosis of abnormally adherent placenta increta or percreta (see below), and when bleeding cannot be controlled with the medical and mechanical methods described above, immediate laparotomy should be undertaken.

6.4.8.2 Partial Placental Retention
A poorly contracted uterus or recurrent episodes of uterine atony should lead to the suspicion of partial placental retention. Re-evaluation of the placenta will usually help to establish the diagnosis, but transabdominal ultrasound is required to confirm it. Uterine curettage should be performed to remove the remaining placental fragments, under regional or general anaesthesia.

6.4.9 Treatment of Rare Causes of Postpartum Haemorrhage

6.4.9.1 Uterine Inversion
Uterine inversion is a very rare but potentially life-threatening situation. It can be diagnosed by vaginal examination, with the inverted uterine fundus found in the uterine cavity (partial inversion), in the vagina (complete inversion) or even in the exterior. The placenta may still be attached to the uterus, and in these situations bleeding may be less intense. Sudden hypotension, pallor and bradycardia occur frequently with uterine inversion, caused by neurogenic shock due to traction on the uterine ligaments. Profuse haemorrhage and hypovolemic shock usually follow. **Manual replacement** should be immediately attempted, before the cervix causes congestion of the inverted fundus, making the procedure increasingly difficult. Continuous pressure is applied around the inverted fundus to push it up through the cervical ring, and this may require 2–3 min. If unsuccessful, medications should be administered for **uterine relaxation** (Table 6.3) and the manoeuvre reattempted. A further reattempt can be made in the operating theatre under general anaesthesia

Table 6.3 Uterine relaxants

Nitroglycerine in slow intravenous bolus (50–100 µg IV slowly)
1 vial of 5 ml (5 mg/ml) in 500 ml of saline. Slow intravenous injection of 1–2 ml (50–100 µg) with continuous monitoring of blood pressure
Salbutamol in intravenous perfusion (125 µg at 25 µ/min)
1 vial of 1 ml (0.5 mg/ml) in 100 ml of saline in intravenous perfusion pump at 300 ml/h during 5 min

with halogenated agents. If the placenta remains attached to the uterine fundus, no efforts should be made to remove it at this stage. Manual removal can be attempted after the uterine fundus is replaced.

Unless reversal is quickly obtained, a prompt decision to undergo **laparotomy** under general anaesthesia with halogenated agents should be taken. Manual repositioning can then be reattempted, but if the cervical constriction ring is too rigid, a posterior vertical incision on this ring usually allows passage of the uterine fundus, after which the incision is closed. After repositioning the uterus, prolonged uterine contracture should be stimulated with an uterotonic agent (Table 6.2).

6.4.9.2 Uterine Rupture

This diagnosis should be considered when bleeding persists in spite of medical and mechanical treatments of uterine atony, particularly when there is a history of previous caesarean section or other surgery involving the myometrium. Digital exploration of the uterine cavity via the vaginal route may identify the wall defect, but the diagnosis is usually only established at laparotomy. Surgical management of uterine rupture is considered in Sect. 2.4.5.

6.4.9.3 Abnormally Adherent Placenta

Management of abnormally adherent placenta when it is diagnosed before labour allows planning of delivery and is beyond the aim of this book. This section refers to the acute management of undiagnosed abnormally adherent placenta at the time of caesarean section or during the third stage of labour. Because these situations are relatively rare, there is little scientific evidence on which to base decisions. Two different clinical situations may be encountered. The first is the suspicion of deep myometrial, peritoneal or adjacent organ invasion at the time of caesarean section, before the uterus is incised. In these cases, confirmation of placental location should be made by intraoperative ultrasound, and the uterine incision needs to avoid the placental bed. After the fetus is delivered, no attempt should be made to extract the placenta. If haemorrhage is minimal and the haemodynamic condition is stable, several approaches may be taken, depending on the patient's desire for future fertility. For patients desiring more children or when these desires are unknown (i.e. patients under general anaesthesia), **partial resection of the uterine wall *en bloc* with the placenta** may be attempted if subsequent closure is judged to be anatomically possible. The alternative is to **leave the placenta *in situ***, ligate the umbilical cord with an absorbable suture close to the placenta and close the uterus in an attempt of expectant management. This option is associated with important haemorrhagic and infectious morbidity, as well as prolonged surveillance, but with careful follow-up has a very low mortality. For patients who do not desire to remain fertile, **peripartum hysterectomy** may be an option when important adjacent organs are not involved in placental invasion. When there is important involvement of adjacent organs or when the expertise for a peripartum hysterectomy is not available, it is preferable to leave the placenta **in situ** and attempt expectant management, even if this results in hysterectomy at a later date. With heavy bleeding and/or a haemodynamically unstable patient, the surgical alternatives described above need to be decided quickly. It is well to remember that definite treatment can be deferred to a later time, and haemorrhage control is the main priority in these situations. Uterine and vaginal packing with gauze, balloon tamponade, B-Lynch sutures, Hayman sutures, uterine and internal iliac artery ligation have all been reported to be successful in a small number of cases. Haemostatic sutures of the placental bed may also be successful in limited areas.

6.4.9.4 Maternal Bleeding Disorders

Several maternal bleeding disorders may be responsible for or may aggravate other causes of postpartum haemorrhage. The detailed description of these conditions is beyond the aims of this chapter, but they are usually managed in collaboration with a haematologist and the hospital blood bank.

6.4.10 Postpartum Haemorrhage at Caesarean Section

Postpartum haemorrhage is more frequent at caesarean section, and it is also easier to quantify blood loss in these situations. Uterine atony remains the most frequent cause, and treatment is not substantially different to that used in vaginal deliveries, involving similar support of maternal circulation/oxygenation and uterotonic agents as first-line treatment (Table 6.2). However, because there is direct access to the uterus, some procedures need to be adapted. Localised uterine atony may benefit from intramyometrial injection of oxytocin, sulprostone and/or carboprost. Bimanual uterine compression is substituted by internal uterine compression, and balloon tamponade can still be performed, but the balloon is usually introduced transabdominally. Compression sutures (Fig. 6.4) are used more frequently, because of ease of access, and they can be combined with balloon tamponade, a procedure that some refer to as the "sandwich technique". Uterine embolisation is seldom employed, because the required equipment is usually unavailable in an operating theatre. Birth canal injuries should still be considered as a possible cause of haemorrhage, particularly when caesarean section was performed during the second stage of labour and/or when there was a difficult fetal extraction.

6.5 Clinical Records and Litigation Issues

It is important to document the names of the healthcare professionals who were summoned, when they were called and when they arrived, which medication and manoeuvres were performed and when and by whom. Inadequate documentation may cause problems when there is medicolegal litigation, and it is therefore helpful to use a structured pro forma for accurate record keeping.

A frank explanation of the situation to the patient and her closest family by an experienced member of the team is also required at the earliest available opportunity.

MANAGEMENT OF POSTPARTUM HEMORRHAGE DUE TO ATONY

Anticipate the situation	Increase hemorrhage evaluation, monitor HR+BP	☐
Clearly verbalise the diagnosis		☐
Ask for help	Two midwives, senior obstetrician, anesthetist	☐
PPH diagnosed	Rapid evaluation of the cause	☐
	External uterine massage	☐
	Catheterise vein with 14-16G and start crystalloids	☐
	Monitoring - BP, HR, O_2 sat, ECG, consciousness	☐
	Oxygen by mask at 30%, 10-15 l/min	☐
	Head down position/elevation of the legs	☐
	Catheterise bladder and measure urine output	☐
	Oxytocin IV in treatment dose	☐
Major PPH diagnosed	Catheterise second vein with 14-16G	☐
	Bimanual uterine compression	☐
	Blood analysis for Hg, coagulation, cross-matching	☐
	Re-evaluate cause	☐
	Rectal misoprostol	☐
	Consider sulprostone or carboprost	☐
	Consider colloids	☐
	Consider blood products - contact hematologist	☐
	Maintain body temperature	☐
	Consider balloon tamponade	☐
	Consider uterine artery embolization (if available)	☐
Decide surgery	Call operating theatre and transfer	☐
	Compression sutures (B-Lynch, Hayman, Pereira)	☐
	Progressive uterine devascularisation	☐
	Consider internal iliac artery ligation	☐
	Consider peripartum hysterectomy	☐
Clinical records	People called, at what time, and when they arrived	☐
	Decisions taken, when and by whom	☐
	Procedures performed, when and by whom	☐

Suggested Reading

Abdel-Aleem H, Hofmeyr GJ, El-Sonoosy E (2006) Uterine massage and postpartum blood loss. Int J Gynecol Obstet 93:238–239

B-Lynch C, Keith L, Lalonde A, Karoshi M (eds) (2006) A textbook of postpartum hemorrhage, 1st edn. Sapiens Publishing, Duncow

Chandraharan E, Arulkumaran S (2008) Surgical aspects of postpartum hemorrhage. Best Pract Res Clin Obstet Gynaecol 22:1089–1102

Ramanathana G, Arulkumaran S (2006) Postpartum hemorrhage. Curr Obstet Gynaecol 16:6–13

Royal College of Obstetricians and Gynaecologists (2009) Prevention and management of postpartum hemorrhage (green-top guideline no. 52). RCOG Press, London

Royal College of Obstetricians and Gynaecologists (2011) Placenta praevia, placenta praevia accrete and vasa praevia: diagnosis and management (green-top guideline no. 27). RCOG Press, London

Maternal Cardiorespiratory Arrest 7

7.1 Definition, Incidence and Main Risk Factors

Maternal cardiorespiratory arrest is estimated to occur in 0.003 % of pregnancies and manifests by **loss of consciousness** and **central cyanosis**. There are a number of possible aetiologies for this event (Table 7.1), but in high-resource countries, pulmonary thromboembolism and amniotic fluid embolism are among the leading causes. A detailed description of the maternal conditions that may lead to cardiorespiratory arrest is beyond the aim of this book, so this chapter will focus on the acute management of the situation and the initial treatment of the two most frequent causes.

Table 7.1 Major causes of maternal cardiorespiratory arrest

Obstetric complications	Major obstetric haemorrhage (abruption, uterine rupture, postpartum haemorrhage)
	Amniotic fluid embolism
Anaesthetic complications	High spinal anaesthesia
	Pulmonary aspiration of gastric contents
	Toxicity of local anaesthetic agents
Medical complications	Pulmonary thromboembolism
	Myocardial infarction
	Aortic dissection
	Peripartum cardiomyopathy
	Anaphylaxis
	Sepsis/septic shock
	Air embolus

© Springer International Publishing Switzerland 2017
D. Ayres-de-Campos, *Obstetric Emergencies*,
DOI 10.1007/978-3-319-41656-4_7

7.2 Consequences

Maternal cardiorespiratory arrest is associated with a high incidence of **maternal deaths** and **long-term neurological sequelae**. It is also associated with important **perinatal mortality** and **long-term neurological sequelae** for the child. Anticipation of the problem and early recognition allow prompt resuscitation and other support measures that have a profound impact on maternal and fetal prognosis.

7.3 Diagnosis

Maternal cardiorespiratory arrest manifests by loss of consciousness and central cyanosis. **Absence of respiratory movements** and **lack of a carotid pulse** confirm the diagnosis. The maternal **electrocardiogram** may display a continuous line representing **asystole**, or there may be **ventricular fibrillation, ventricular tachycardia** or any other type of **electric activity without a carotid pulse**.

7.4 Clinical Management

Whatever the cause of maternal cardiorespiratory arrest, the initial response is similar and involves the **support of maternal oxygenation and circulation** and **rapid delivery of the fetus if the situation does not revert within 4 min**. When both an anaesthetist and an obstetrician are present, the responsibility for these two aspects is usually divided among them. In the remaining cases, the most senior healthcare professional needs to take charge of the whole situation. Management of cardiorespiratory arrest occurring after delivery does not differ significantly from that occurring in the non-pregnant woman and is beyond the aim of this chapter.

7.4.1 Anticipating the Situation

The occurrence of sudden maternal **shortness of breath** (dyspnoea and tachypnoea) associated with **central cyanosis** suggests a serious respiratory complication that may be followed by cardiorespiratory arrest. When such symptoms occur, the woman should be placed in **left lateral safety position** (Fig. 7.1), and several of the aspects considered below can be anticipated, including **maternal and fetal monitoring, vein catheterisation, summoning of appropriate staff** and **collection of equipment** that may later be required (emergency trolley).

7.4.2 Clearly Verbalising the Diagnosis

It is important that all members of the healthcare team are aware of the diagnosis of maternal cardiorespiratory arrest, and therefore this needs to be clearly verbalised.

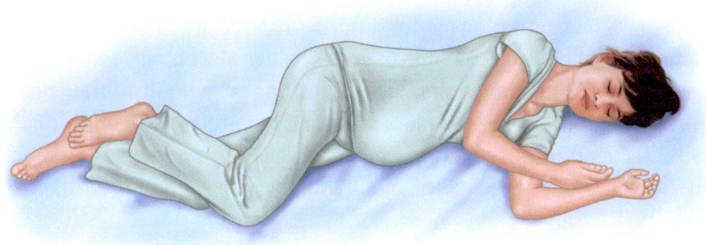

Fig. 7.1 Left lateral safety position

7.4.3 Asking for Help

One of the first measures should be to summon urgently **at least two midwives**, a **senior obstetrician**, an **anaesthetist** and the **hospital resuscitation team**. As stated above, the presence of an anaesthetist guarantees a safer management of respiratory and circulatory functions, as well as basic fluid balance. Care is however needed to maintain good communication between both sides at all times, so that there is coordinated management of the situation.

7.4.4 Maternal Monitoring

When cardiorespiratory arrest occurs in a hospital environment, maternal monitoring is a priority for objective assessment and response to treatment, so continuous evaluation of **heart rate**, **oxygen saturation and electrocardiography** should be started promptly and the **blood pressure** measured at least every 5–10 min.

7.4.5 Support of Maternal Oxygenation and Circulation

7.4.5.1 A (Airway): Guarantee the Patency of the Airway
To guarantee the patency of the airway, the patient should be turned onto her back, the head tilted backwards, the chin lifted and the **mouth opened and inspected for objects** that may cause obstruction. Secretions may be aspirated if abundant and a **Mayo tube** temporarily introduced to prevent the tongue from occluding the airway, if endotracheal intubation cannot be immediately performed.

7.4.5.2 B (Breathing): Maintain Oxygen Supply to the Lungs
To maintain oxygen supply to the lungs, **ventilation with a bag-valve mask** should be immediately started at 15 cycles/min, using **100 % oxygen** and **15 l/min**, and thereafter adapting according to oxygen saturation levels, which should be kept over 90 %. After obtaining the necessary material, **early endotracheal intubation**

should be performed to improve the efficacy of ventilation and prevent aspiration of gastric contents. The ventilation cycles described above are maintained. If available, capnography should be used to confirm correct tube placement, as well as the adequacy of ventilation and cardiac massage. **Pulmonary auscultation** is necessary to evaluate proper endotracheal tube placement and the presence of additional respiratory sounds. As soon as possible, arterial blood gas sampling should be performed to evaluate whether the objective of maintaining partial pressure of oxygen above 60 mmHg is being achieved.

7.4.5.3 C (Circulation): Cardiac Massage and Vein Catheterisation

With maternal loss of consciousness and an absent carotid pulse, **immediate external cardiac massage** should be started, independently of whether or not cardiac activity is detected on the electrocardiogram. A **hard board** should be placed underneath the woman, and if pregnancy is above 20 weeks, a hard object is placed under this board to create a **30° left tilt** (Fig. 7.2 – left). The objective is to avoid aorto-caval compression by the pregnant uterus and the resulting decreased venous return from the lower limbs. If this is not immediately available, an alternative is to shift the abdomen laterally and **displace the uterus to the left** (Fig. 7.2 – centre).

Cardiac massage is performed by placing two interlocked hands on the inferior portion of the patient's sternum and with the arms fully stretched, applying rhythmic compressions at 100 cycles per minute, depressing the sternum by about 5 cm (Fig. 7.2 – right). There is ample evidence that appropriately applied cardiac massage causes respiratory movements, so this should be the prioritised manoeuvre if no one is available to guarantee ventilation. Cardiac massage is only stopped for brief seconds every 2 min, to re-evaluate cardiac rhythm and the carotid pulse. The procedure is only abandoned when an adequate cardiac rhythm and pulse are detected, or when death is declared.

As soon as possible, **vein catheterisation with a large bore catheter** (14G or 16G) should be carried out. In all situations of cardiorespiratory arrest, **adrenaline 1 mg in intravenous bolus** should be given as soon as the venous catheter is in place and repeated on alternate 2 min cycles of cardiac massage. After the first bolus is given, blood should be collected for complete blood

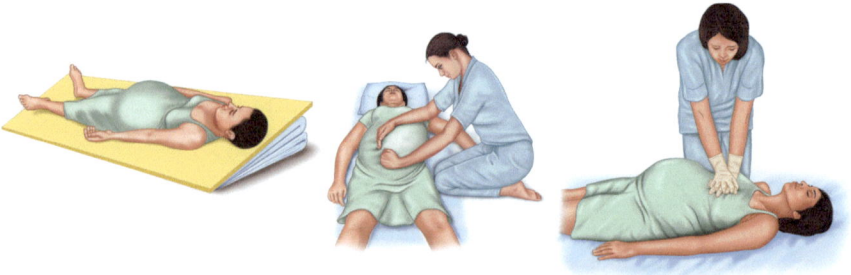

Fig. 7.2 Hard board and 30° left tilt (*left*), left lateral abdominal displacement (*centre*), positioning of the body and hands for external cardiac massage (*right*)

count, electrolytes, liver and renal function, coagulation studies and cross-matching. **Fluid replacement with crystalloids** (saline, Ringer's lactate) should follow.

7.4.6 Bladder Catheterisation and Measurement of Urinary Output

Bladder catheterisation should be performed to measure urinary output and fluid balance adapted to maintain the latter above 30 ml/h.

7.4.7 Fetal Monitoring

At viable gestational ages, continuous cardiotocography should be performed quickly started, although the measure should ideally anticipate cardiorespiratory arrest (see Chap. 2).

7.4.8 *In Situ* Caesarean Section

When pregnancy is above 20 weeks and there is no reversal after 4 min of cardiorespiratory arrest, *in situ* **caesarean section** is indicated to improve the chances of maternal resuscitation and to avoid the consequences of prolonged acute fetal hypoxia in viable pregnancies. Moving the patient to the operating theatre is not recommended in these situations, as it delays the procedure, so caesarean section should be performed at the site of arrest. Because of reduced circulation with external cardiac massage, bleeding is usually minimal, and no anaesthesia is required as the patient is unconscious. The abdomen is previously disinfected, the abdominal skin is opened with a scalpel, and fetal extraction is quickly carried out, as in normal caesarean delivery. Cardiac massage and assisted ventilation are continued throughout the whole process. After the fetus is delivered, the surgical procedure can be completed at a slower pace, and more attention should again be given to maternal resuscitation.

7.4.9 Defribrillatory Rhythms

When **ventricular fibrillation** and **ventricular tachycardia without pulse** are detected, electric defibrillation is frequently successful in reverting cardiorespiratory arrest. A **200 J biphasic** or **360 J monophasic** shock should be applied (Fig. 7.3). Before this, the team must temporarily stop cardiac massage and ventilation, remove the oxygen source and step away from the patient and her bed. If there is no reversal after the first shock, a second shock is indicated. If the abnormal rhythm persists after the second shock, **adrenaline 1 mg in intravenous bolus** should be administered on alternate cardiac massage cycles and a third shock applied. If the rhythm persists after the third shock, **amiodarone 300 mg in intravenous bolus** is administered.

Fig. 7.3 Location of the electric pads for defibrillation

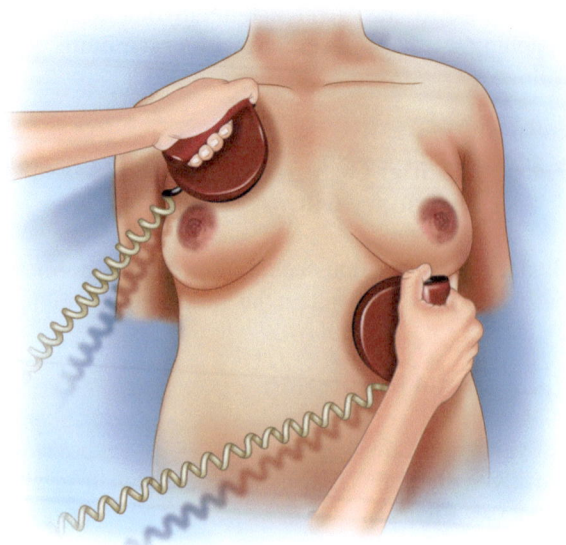

7.4.10 After Cardiorespiratory Arrest Reverses

If there is reversal of cardiorespiratory arrest, the situation requires re-evaluation in a more serene context.

7.4.10.1 Hypotension
When there is sustained hypotension, **ephedrine**, **dopamine**, **dobutamine** and **colloids** need to be considered. The objective is to maintain mean arterial pressure above 65 mmHg and urine output above 30 ml/h. In addition to these, blood products, including red blood cells, fresh frozen plasma, cryoprecipitate and platelets, may be required, particularly when there is disseminated intravascular coagulation and persistent haemorrhage (see Chap. 6).

7.4.10.2 Termination of Pregnancy
The decision to terminate pregnancy after reversal of cardiorespiratory arrest has occurred depends on gestational age and on the clinical stability of the situation. A caesarean section is usually indicated if pregnancy is above 34 weeks and the patient is haemodynamically stable. At earlier gestational ages, management depends mostly on the underlying cause, on haemodynamic stability and on the results of cardiotocography and ultrasound. In some cases, it may be justifiable to maintain vigilance or to wait 48 h for the effect of a corticosteroid course.

7.4.10.3 Monitoring in an Intensive Care Unit

After the initial stabilisation, patients require transfer to an intensive care unit for closer observation, where arterial catheterisation with invasive blood pressure monitoring, serial blood gas analysis, central venous catheterisation and pressure monitoring may be required.

7.4.10.4 Maintain Body Temperature

Low body temperature contributes to peripheral hypoperfusion and to tissue damage. This can be reduced by maintaining normal body temperature and by administering previously warmed fluids.

7.4.10.5 Looking for an Underlying Cause

After the initial response to maternal cardiorespiratory arrest, further evaluation of the underlying cause should be carried out as soon as the patient is stabilised (Table 7.1). It is sometimes possible to suspect the diagnosis from analysis of clinical records and/or from a patient history obtained from a relative. **Chest X-ray**, **d-dimers**, **electrocardiogram**, **echocardiogram** and **ventilation/perfusion scan** may be useful in establishing the definite diagnosis.

7.4.11 Pulmonary Thromboembolism

Pulmonary thromboembolism has a fatality rate of 1 % and is one of the leading causes of maternal mortality in high-resource countries. The association of shortness of breath, tachypnoea, cough and pleuritic chest pain is very suggestive, but the clinical presentation is variable. The presence of risk factors (Table 7.2) contributes to the suspicion. Diminished respiratory sounds on auscultation are only found in 50 % of cases, and oxygen saturation is usually low.

Table 7.2 Risk factors for pulmonary thromboembolism

Pre-existing medical complications	Cardiac disease
	Hypertension, diabetes mellitus, obesity
	Systemic lupus erythematosus
	Smoking
	Thrombophilia – protein S or C deficiencies
	Previous thromboembolic disease
Pregnancy complications	Multiple pregnancy
	Hyperemesis/dehydration
	Antepartum or postpartum haemorrhage
	Prolonged labour
	Infection
	Caesarean section and instrumental vaginal delivery
	Artificial placental extraction or curettage

Table 7.3 Therapeutic doses of low molecular weight heparin (according to early pregnancy weight)

	<50 kg	50–69 kg	70–89 kg	>90 kg
Enoxaparin	40 mg 12/12 h	60 mg 12/12 h	80 mg 12/12 h	100 mg 12/12 h
Dalteparin	5000 IU 12/12 h	6000 IU 12/12 h	8000 IU 12/12 h	10,000 IU 12/12 h
Tinzaparin	175 units/kg once daily			

Although the definite diagnosis requires a high degree of certainty, as it implies prolonged therapy and increased vigilance, a reasonable suspicion should be enough to initiate anticoagulant therapy (Table 7.3), except when there is an absolute contraindication, such as hepatic insufficiency or a high risk of bleeding, as delaying treatment will strongly condition outcome. **Low molecular weight heparin** does not cross the placenta, is administered subcutaneously and does not require close monitoring of coagulation results, so it is usually the preferred method of treatment. The alternative is heparin, administered intravenously at 80 units/kg for 12 h (maximum of 10,000 units), followed by a perfusion of 18 units/kg/h (maximum of 2200 units/h). Low molecular weight and unfractionated heparin have an equivalent efficacy, but the latter requires coagulation tests 6 h after the loading dose, or after any dose change, and thereafter at least daily. In these situations, activated partial thromboplastin time should be kept 1.5–2.5 times the basal value, and platelet count should be monitored every other day. Treatment should be continued until the diagnosis is excluded.

Arterial blood gas analysis will frequently reveal hypoxaemia, and metabolic acidosis may also be present. The **chest X-ray** is normal in about 50 % of the cases, but several non-specific changes may appear, such as cardiac enlargement, small opacities, atelectasis, pleural effusion or pulmonary oedema. This exam is also important to exclude other diseases, such as pneumonia and pneumothorax. **D-dimers** may be increased in the absence of thromboembolism, because of increased fibrinolysis during pregnancy and after surgery, but the test has a high negative predictive value, as normal values almost completely exclude the diagnosis. The **electrocardiogram** usually displays non-specific changes, such as sinus tachycardia, but it is also important for other diagnoses. **Doppler ultrasound of the lower limbs** is useful to establish the diagnosis of deep vein thrombosis, which predisposes to pulmonary thromboembolism and has an identical treatment. **Ventilation/perfusion scan** is commonly used in pregnant women to establish the definite diagnosis of pulmonary thromboembolism, as it carries less risks of radiation than **computerised tomography pulmonary angiography**, but the latter has the highest accuracy and may be necessary in some cases.

In severe cases of **massive pulmonary thromboembolism** associated with serious haemodynamic compromise, unfractionated heparin is the treatment of choice, and thrombolytic therapy, thrombus fragmentation, thoracotomy and surgical embolectomy may all need to be considered.

7.4.12 Amniotic Fluid Embolism Syndrome

This syndrome appears to be caused by an anaphylactic reaction to amniotic fluid or to another unknown substance that gains access to the maternal circulation. It occurs

Table 7.4 Risk factors for amniotic fluid embolism

Advanced maternal age
High parity
Induction of labour
Multiple pregnancy
Caesarean section
Cervical laceration
Uterine rupture

more frequently during labour or in the 30 min that follow, but may also arise during pregnancy, particularly in association with second and third trimester abortion or in the 4 h after delivery.

It is reported to occur in 0.002 % of all pregnancies, but sub-diagnosis is likely. In high-resource countries, it accounts for approximately 10 % of all direct maternal deaths. The common features are **pulmonary arteriolar constriction** followed by **left ventricular failure**. The resulting symptoms and signs are **profound hypotension, shortness of breath, central cyanosis, loss of consciousness, seizures** and **cardiorespiratory arrest**. In a second phase, there is **thromboplastin release** into the maternal circulation, caused by activation of the coagulation cascade, with resulting **disseminated intravascular coagulation** and **postpartum haemorrhage**. The main risk factors are displayed in Table 7.4.

Maternal mortality varies between 13 and 61 %, and about 10 % of survivors develop neurological sequelae. Perinatal mortality affects 9–44 % of cases, and almost 50 % of survivors will have long-term sequelae.

Currently, there is no gold standard test for this syndrome, so the diagnosis is based on suggestive clinical features and the exclusion of other diagnoses such as eclampsia, high anaesthetic blockade, systemic toxicity by local anaesthetics, gas embolism, anaphylactic reaction to medications, peripartum cardiomyopathy and myocardial infarction. Even when there is maternal death, findings at autopsy are unspecific. Chest X-ray, electrocardiogram and ventilation/perfusion scan should be considered to exclude other possible causes.

Likewise, there is no specific treatment for amniotic fluid embolism, beyond the support measures described above, and correction of ensuing complications. Some authors propose the use of 500 mg hydrocortisone IV every 6 h, to reduce the anaphylactic response, but there is insufficient proof of benefit. Anticipation of postpartum haemorrhage is an essential part of treatment.

7.5 Clinical Records and Litigation Issues

It is important to document the names of the healthcare professionals who were summoned, when they were called and when they arrived, which medication and manoeuvres were performed, when and by whom. These aspects may be crucial if there is medicolegal litigation.

A frank explanation of the situation to the patient and her closest family needs to be given by an experienced member of the team who was involved in management. The overall attitude and the words of healthcare professionals remain for a long time in people's memories, associated with such difficult moments. Thoughtless words, a rushed or cold attitude will frequently be remembered as negative experiences, while kindness and concern will usually be an important source of comfort.

MANAGEMENT OF MATERNAL CARDIORESPIRATORY ARREST

Anticipate the situation	Left lateral safety position	☐
	Start maternal + fetal monitoring (see below)	☐
	Catheterise vein with 14-16G and start crystalloids	☐
	Place emergency trolley nearby	☐
Clearly verbalise the diagnosis		☐
Ask for help	2 midwives, obstetrician, anesthetist, resus. team	☐
Maternal monitoring	BP, HR, O_2 sat, ECG, consciousness	☐
Airway + breathing	Turn on back, inspect mouth	☐
	Mayo tube + bag ventilation 100% O_2, 15 l/min	☐
	Endotracheal intubation + bag ventilation	☐
	Pulmonary auscultation	☐
Circulation	Hard board + 30° tilt or abdominal displacement	☐
	External cardiac massage 100/min, 5 cm	☐
	Stop every 2 min to evaluate rhythm + pulse	☐
	Vein catheterisation 14-16G + crystalloids	☐
	Adrenalin 1 g IV on alternate cycles	☐
	If vent. fibrillation or tachycardia no pulse → shock	☐
	Amiodarone 300 mg after 3rd shock	☐
	Blood count + elect + liver/renal + coag. + match	☐
	Bladder catheterisation + urine output	☐
Fetal monitoring	Continuous CTG	☐
If no reversal by 4 min	*In situ* c-section	☐
After stabilisation	Re-evaluation of the cause	☐
Clinical records	People called, at what time, and when they arrived	☐
	Decisions taken, when and by whom	☐
	Procedures performed, when and by whom	☐

Suggested Reading

Benson MD, Kobayashi H, Silver RK, Oi H, Greenberger PA, Terao T (2001) Immunologic studies in presumed amniotic fluid embolism. Obstet Gynecol 97:510–514

Clark SL, Howkins GDV, Dudley DA, Dildy GA, Porter TF (1999) Amniotic fluid embolism: analysis of a national registry. Am J Obstet Gynecol 172:1158–1169

Conde-Agudelo A, Romero R (2009) Amniotic fluid embolism: an evidence-based review. Am J Obstet Gynecol 201(5):445.e1–445.e13

Greer I (2001) The acute management of venous thromboembolism in pregnancy. Curr Opin Obstet Gynecol 13:569–575

James A (2008) Thromboembolism in pregnancy: recurrence risks, prevention and management. Curr Opin Obstet Gynecol 20:550–556

Knight M, Tuffnell D, Brockelhurst P, Spark P, Kurinczuk JJ, on behalf of the UJ Obstetric Surveillance System (2010) Incidence and risk factors for amniotic fluid embolism. Obstet Gynecol 115:910–917

Krivak T, Zorn KK (2007) Venous thromboembolism in obstetrics and gynecology. Obstet Gynecol 109:761–777

Royal College of Obstetricians and Gynaecologists (2007) Thromboembolic disease in pregnancy and the puerperium: acute management (Green-top guideline no. 28). RCOG Press, London

Royal College of Obstetricians and Gynaecologists (2009) Reducing the risk of thrombosis and embolism during pregnancy and the puerperium (Green-top guideline no. 37). RCOG Press, London

Weiwen Y, Niugyu Z, Lauxiang Z, Yu L (2000) Study of the diagnosis and management of amniotic fluid embolism: 38 cases of analysis. Obstet Gynecol 95(4 Suppl):38S

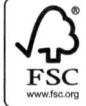

MIX
Papier aus verantwortungsvollen Quellen
Paper from responsible sources
FSC® C105338

If you have any concerns about our products,
you can contact us on
ProductSafety@springernature.com

In case Publisher is established outside the EU,
the EU authorized representative is:
**Springer Nature Customer Service Center GmbH
Europaplatz 3, 69115 Heidelberg, Germany**

Printed by Libri Plureos GmbH
in Hamburg, Germany